Essential Microbiology for Wound Care

Edited by

Valerie Edwards-Jones

Emeritus Professor of Medical Microbiology
School of Healthcare Science
Manchester Metropolitan University, UK

Clinical Director,
MelBec Microbiology Ltd, Haslingden
Rossendale, Lancashire, UK

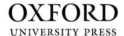

OXFORD
UNIVERSITY PRESS

OXFORD
UNIVERSITY PRESS

Great Clarendon Street, Oxford, OX2 6DP,
United Kingdom

Oxford University Press is a department of the University of Oxford.
It furthers the University's objective of excellence in research, scholarship,
and education by publishing worldwide. Oxford is a registered trade mark of
Oxford University Press in the UK and in certain other countries

First Edition published in 2016

Impression: 3

Published in the United States of America by Oxford University Press
198 Madison Avenue, New York, NY 10016, United States of America

British Library Cataloguing in Publication Data

Data available

Library of Congress Control Number: 2015944342

ISBN 978–0–19–871600–6

Printed and bound by
CPI Group (UK) Ltd, Croydon, CR0 4YY

Essential Microbiology for Wound Care

Foreword by Gregory Schultz

Optimal care of both acute and chronic wounds requires effective management of the bacterial bioburden, yet many wound care providers (physicians, nurses, and podiatrists) have limited training in basic aspects of microbiology, which reduces their effectiveness in selecting and using advanced wound care products. This 'gap in their knowledge base' can result in inconsistent or suboptimal wound care that can lead to substantial complications including sepsis or amputations.

Fortunately, the new text 'Essential Microbiology for Wound Care' edited by *Valerie Edwards-Jones*, Emeritus Professor of Medical Microbiology, and former Director of Research at Manchester Metropolitan University, UK, is a major aid in filling this knowledge gap for wound care providers. Professor Edwards-Jones has enlisted a very distinguished list of contributors who are leaders in their areas of microbiology and clinical wound care. The list of topics spans the spectrum from the basic science of microbiology to clinical translation of the key principles into effective wound care. These include chapters on new developments in understanding bacterial biofilms, advances in antimicrobial agents, descriptions of antimicrobial dressing used in wound care, strategies to reduce wound infection and to optimize treatments for infected wounds.

Busy clinicians will find the structure of the chapters to be very 'user-friendly'. Each chapter includes a concise list of the important information covered in the chapter and a summary of the key facts discussed and written in terms the non-microbiologist can readily understand.

This new text is highly recommended for both new and experienced wound care clinicians because it effectively bridges the knowledge gap that often exists between understanding basic microbiology and effective translation into prevention of wound infection or effective clinical management of wound bioburden.

Professor Gregory Schultz, PhD
Department of Obstetrics and Gynecology
Institute for Wound Research
University of Florida, USA

Foreword by Sue Bale

The publication of this book is so timely with the growth in discussion and debate surrounding the importance of infection, microbial resistance, and the challenges associated with developing new antibiotics and alternative therapies. The risk of wound infection is a constant clinical challenge, which can delay healing for individual patients, affect their quality of life, whilst adversely impacting on health systems' economies. The early detection of infection by deploying the best diagnostics will help clinical staff to move quickly to treat infection, thus reducing its economic and personal costs.

Our knowledge of the role of biofilms in wounds has emerged over the past 10 years, alongside the negative effects of biofilms throughout other sites in the human body. Effective recognition, detection and management of biofilms in wounds that is underpinned by sound knowledge, and the clinical experiences of experts will be key to providing the best clinical care possible for patients. If we can bring together the knowledge and experience of expert wound healing professionals with the research of laboratory and clinical scientists then we will be well on the way to transforming recalcitrant, non-healing wounds into healed wounds.

At a practical level many wounds require a dressing to manage exudates, drainage, pain, and cosmesis. When infection and bacterial burden is also present, decisions about which of the many dressings to use can be challenging. Clinical staff need to be aware of the indications of use, functions, application and contraindications of these dressings if they are to effectively utilize them to effectively manage infection and bacterial burden.

As science moves forward and progress is made to improve interventions for patients, it is essential that these discoveries are brought together and assimilated and then compared and contrasted with existing treatments. 'Essential Microbiology for Wound Care' does this, garnering the expertise of researchers and clinical leaders, who as authors have contributed to this text.

This book guides clinical staff in managing the broad range of clinical challenges that relate to bacteria and wounds and it is hugely relevant to these healthcare professionals. The effects of applying the knowledge, information, and guidance contained within this book will no doubt help to prevent complications associated with microbes, which can be serious and life threatening.

Professor Sue Bale, OBE
FRCN, PhD, BA, RGN, NDN, RHV, PG Dip, Dip N
Research and Development Director
Aneurin Bevan University Health Board
St Cadoc's Hospital
Newport, UK

Preface

This book is aimed at the wound care practitioner and hopefully will give an understanding of the role of microorganisms in the healing process and how colonization and infection can impede this.

The various chapters describe fundamental principles of microbiology and most examples are focused around wound care. However, in order to ensure full understanding, alternative examples are also used to emphasize a particular principle.

The book is written in such a style that certain aspects can be revisited in order to aid understanding of some microbiological problems. The objectives of each chapter are listed and throughout the chapters key important points are highlighted, as are interesting facts.

All the authors are experts in their own fields and they have written their chapters to help you understand the full impact of microbiology and wound care.

Enjoy reading . . .

Contents

List of Contributors

Rose Cooper
Professor of Microbiology
Cardiff School of Health Sciences
Cardiff Metropolitan
University, UK

Geoff Edwards-Jones
Director, Essential Microbiology
Ltd, UK

Valerie Edwards-Jones
Emeritus Professor of Medical
Microbiology
School of Healthcare Science
Manchester Metropolitan
University, UK

Clinical Director, MelBec
Microbiology Ltd, Haslingden
Rossendale, Lancashire, UK

Madeleine Flanagan
Principal Lecturer
Postgraduate Medicine
School of Life and Medical
Sciences
University of Hertfordshire, UK

Jacqui Fletcher
Clinical Strategy Director
Welsh Wound Innovation Centre
Rhondda Cynon Taf, UK

Keith Harding
Professor Keith Harding CBE
FRCGP, FRCP, FRCS, FLSW

Dean of Clinical Innovation
Head of Wound Healing Research
Unit (WHRU)
School of Medicine
Cardiff University, UK

Medical Director
Welsh Wound Innovation Centre
Ynysmaerdy, UK

Martin Kiernan
Richard Wells Research Centre
College of Nursing, Midwifery
and Healthcare
The University of West London, UK

Chris Roberts
Principal Consultant
Clinical Resolutions Ltd
Hull, UK

Alastair Richards
Clinical Research Fellow
School of Medicine
Cardiff University, UK

Richard White
Professor of Tissue Viability
Institute of Health & Society
University of Worcester, UK

Chapter 1

Introduction

Valerie Edwards-Jones

Introduction to wound microbiology

Prevention and treatment of infection in wounds is not a new science. In fact, medical information on wound care was documented on clay tablets discovered in Mesopotamia dating back to around 2500 BC. Other medical information found on papyrus in Egypt also gives an insight into how medicine was practised (Forrest 1982). People have always dressed wounds, using a variety of substances and methods, with the prime aim to promote quick healing of the injury and to prevent infection. Many other treatment strategies for wound care have been passed down the centuries through folk lore and other documentation.

Hippocrates, some 2400 years ago, wrote of the use of boiled or filtered water for washing wounds, application of tar (an early antiseptic), and the use of compresses for dressing wounds, using oil, wine, or vinegar (Elliot 1964). Reviews of ancient literature reveal that various other medicines have been tried alongside a variety of surgical techniques. Early surgeons in the thirteenth and fourteenth centuries recognized that the formation of pus in a wound would be problematic for wound healing along with dead and decaying tissue, and its removal was widely practised (**early debridement**). In addition, different ointments would be applied to the wound to eradicate any poisons that may have accumulated in the wound (**antiseptics**). In current practice, wound care still uses the basic premise of cleaning, debridement, and dressing of the wound, following whatever surgical intervention is required. This is very important from a microbiological perspective. Dead and decaying tissue must be removed since bacteria will use this to grow and multiply in the wound bed, producing toxins and enzymes that will impede wound healing. Cleansing is also very important to remove accumulation of toxic substances in wound exudate. Cleansing will also facilitate removal of some free-floating bacteria which would otherwise attach to the wound bed and continue to create problems for wound healing. The overall impact of good wound cleansing and debridement is the reduction of organism numbers and removal of nutrients that will allow bacterial growth. A good clean wound bed with low numbers of microorganisms is necessary for the migration of new cells and ultimate wound closure.

Whilst research into wound biology has helped understand a number of reasons why some wounds do not heal, there are still a large number of unknowns and in the last decade the importance of 'biofilms' in wounds has been recognized. The interaction of microorganisms in this form with the host tissues contributes to the chronicity of the wound and prevents healing. How to eradicate these microorganisms will be discussed in later chapters, but how to prevent them is also essential to enable the desired rapid healing. Wounds that remain unhealed for a long time are known to produce worse scarring.

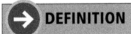 **DEFINITION**

A **biofilm** is an aggregate of microorganisms attached to a surface, encased in a protective matrix.

In addition to research into the biology of wound healing, there has also been a massive increase in the number of wound care products available including novel dressings, such as antimicrobial-impregnated dressings, cleaning agents, and innovative diagnostic tools. Skin substitutes for the burned or traumatized patient are helping to produce a more favourable outcome for the patient in terms of appearance.

In the last two decades, increased numbers of antibiotic-resistant bacteria have been isolated from wounds and although they do not always cause infection in the host their carriage can be a source of infection for other vulnerable groups of patients. If these organisms do cause wound infection in the patient, then the treatment is more difficult as the availability of antibiotics diminishes. The number of new antibiotics to be produced over the next decade is in single figures (Cooke 2004) so as wound care practitioners, alternative methods of preventing and treating wound infection must be reviewed. All wound care practices and associated products used in wound care must be thoroughly evaluated and evidence reported to help improve the outcome for the patient. Also, a full understanding of the interaction of microorganisms with the various stages of wound healing will help us understand how we can best protect the patient from infection or prolonged wound healing.

Wound care places an enormous burden on healthcare services in terms of cost of wound dressings and treatments, nursing care, surgical interventions and emotional impact on the patient. This is compounded when there is an associated infection, or when there is a non-healing chronic wound. Therefore a good understanding of how microorganisms reproduce and cause disease is essential and the appropriate use of antimicrobials and cleansing procedures to reduce microbial load is necessary to diminish this burden on health services.

Microbiology is a very complex subject area and it is hoped that this text will provide wound care professionals with the most practical and applicable information regarding the importance of microbes in wound care, including bacterial, fungal, viral, and parasitic diseases.

What is microbiology?

Microbiology is the study of living organisms that can be so small that they cannot be seen by the naked eye. Microorganisms (bacteria, fungi, viruses, and parasites) vary in size (see Table 1.1) and a variety of different types of microscopes are used to visualize them. The first primitive microscopes were made in the seventeenth century and since then a wide range of microscopes have been developed to help the microbiologist.

FACT

A simple light microscope can magnify an object up to approximately 400 times and is often used to see bacteria, fungi, and parasites. A sophisticated electron microscope, which can magnify up to approximately 10,000 times, is needed to visualize viruses which are about 500–1000 times smaller than bacteria.

Microorganisms are ubiquitous and exist in the air, water, soil, animals, and plants. The human body is covered with microorganisms and generally they do no harm, existing in high numbers in moist areas, for example, the armpits (axilla), groin, and the feet. If we do not wash regularly, they continue to increase in number, break down fatty acids, and start to produce an odour (body odour). They are also found in very high numbers in the bowel and one gram of faeces contains about one million million bacterial cells (10^{12}). It is very easy to transfer organisms from the bowel onto the hands which is why handwashing after toilet use is important. The hands are the commonest vehicle for transferring organisms from one person to the other.

Table 1.1 Comparative sizes of microorganisms

Size	Organism	Observed by
1 m (metre)	Tapeworm	Naked eye
0.5 mm (millimetres)	Scabies	Naked eye/ magnifying lens
10 mm	Threadworms	
1–4 μm (micrometres)	*Staphylococcus* spp. (bacteria)	Light microscope
10–12 μm	*Streptococcus* spp. (bacteria)	
	Pseudomonas spp. (bacteria) Malaria (protozoa)	
1–10 nm (nanometres)	Pox virus	Electron microscope
	Influenza virus	
	Polio virus	

Microorganisms can be beneficial to humans and are used extensively in the food and drink industry as part of the processes used to make bread, cheese, yoghurt, and alcohol. They are integral to natural processes where they break down organic material into nutrients that can be recycled and used by other organisms. However, they can also cause devastating disease in humans, plants, and animals, which creates a huge health burden on society.

Microbiology as a science has expanded greatly over the last 50 years and parallels many of the developments in technology, medicine, and analytical science. Although many traditional methods are still used routinely to identify potential microbes causing infectious disease, a variety of new techniques is being made available. Through the application of these techniques, we are beginning to fully understand some of the issues that have concerned microbiologists for years. These new technologies have allowed a more comprehensive understanding of how we live alongside these microscopic living organisms in health and disease. Detection of important genes within the microbial cell and their regulation at a molecular level can help develop new treatment strategies. In addition, understanding the epidemiology and spread of disease has allowed us to reduce the risk of acquiring infection and vaccination has protected society against some of the most devastating infectious diseases known to humankind. For example, through vaccination, no new cases of smallpox (a viral disease) have been recorded for over 30 years. There have been no cases of bubonic plague (a bacterial disease) in the Western world for a decade, although there are still occasional cases reported in Asia and other developing countries. Prevention and treatment of infection using antimicrobial agents has reduced infection for many and hopefully will continue to do so in years to come, even though antimicrobial resistance is increasing as the microorganisms adapt.

Can all microorganisms cause disease in humans?

There are thousands of different microorganisms, but only about 400 different species of bacteria, fungi, viruses, and parasites cause infection in humans. These are termed 'pathogens' and they possess different properties that allow them to overcome the immune response and develop clinical infection. Such microorganisms are called 'pathogenic' and their ability to cause disease is due to their 'virulence' or 'pathogenicity'.

Microorganisms that do not cause infection are termed 'non-pathogens', that is, they do not possess any properties that allow them to overcome the immune system and cause clinical disease.

Another group of microorganisms may be termed 'opportunistic pathogens' and this means they are capable of causing disease when the host is immunocompromised for whatever reason. An example of an opportunistic infection is when a common skin organism *Staphylococcus epidermidis* (which is part of the normal skin flora) enters the bloodstream through a plastic cannula resulting in bacteraemia.

 KEY POINT

- A **pathogen** is a microorganism capable of invading the body and causing disease.

- A **non-pathogen** is a microorganism not capable of causing disease

- An **opportunistic pathogen** is capable of causing infection in immunocompromised individuals

- A **commensal** is a microorganism that lives in harmony with the host and other microorganisms.

- **Normal flora** are microorganisms frequently found in a particular niche, not causing harm to the host (sometimes termed commensal flora).

An example of a wound pathogen that can cause devastating disease is *Clostridium perfringens* which causes gas gangrene. This infection may result as a complication of a fracture or after surgery. The pathogen, *Clostridium perfringens*, enters the wound (usually following contamination from the bowel) and when there is restricted oxygen, the organism will grow within the wound causing necrosis (gangrene) and gas will be produced within the tissues. As *Clostridium perfringens* grows, it produces a powerful toxin (poison) that kills any cell it attacks (red blood cells, white blood cells, and tissue cells) causing massive tissue destruction.

How humans are protected from infection: the immune system

The immune system is a flexible protection system that protects the human body against invasion by microorganisms. It is not foolproof and many pathogens can overcome the immune defences and cause disease. The immune defence system is broadly divided into the non-specific (innate or natural) system and the specific (adaptive) immune system. If either system is compromised because of poor health, a poor vascular supply, poor nutrition, and so on, then an individual will be more prone to contracting infection or being colonized by microorganisms.

! FACT

The immune system protects people from infection and is broadly divided into two parts: the **non-specific** and the **specific** immune system. The **non-specific** system includes numerous physical mechanisms, such as the inflammation reaction, cough reflex, and skin structure, and physiological factors, enzymes, complement, lactoferrin, mucous, macrophages, and cytokines. The **specific** system is focused on the production of protective antibodies.

What is non-specific immunity?

Many components of this system are normal mechanical and physiological properties of the host, for example, the integrity of the skin, fatty acid secretion, mechanical flushing, ciliary action leading to removal of mucous and debris in the respiratory tract, enzymatic action of lysozyme in tears, complement, phagocytes, and normal flora. If the health of an individual is compromised through surgery, or they have medical devices *in situ*, are at extremes of age, have a poor vascular supply, have uncontrolled diabetes, or other health issues and poor nutrition, then they will be very prone to infection.

One of the most important non-specific events that are responsible for protecting the host is the **inflammation reaction**. There are four major responses observed at the site of infection—pain, heat, redness, and swelling—and although the inflammation reaction occurs in every individual, the responses may vary depending upon the host or the pathogen. Traditional clinical signs of a wound infection are purulent discharge, spreading erythema, pain, and swelling. These are described by Cutting and Harding (1994) and revised by Cutting and White (2006) where symptoms of infection in different wound types are described in more detail. Box 1.1 describes the criteria used to describe an acute wound infection, with additional criteria describing clinical manifestations in a chronic wound.

Box 1.1 Signs and symptoms of a wound infection

Traditional wound infection criteria

- Abscess
- Cellulitis
- Discharge, including serous exudate, with inflammation, sero-purulent, haemo-purulent, and pus.

Additional criteria

- Delayed healing
- Discolouration
- Friable granulation tissue which bleeds easily
- Unexpected pain or tenderness
- Pocketing at the base of the wound
- Bridging of the epithelium or soft tissue
- Abnormal smell.

Source: data from Cutting KF and Harding KG, Criteria for identifying wound infection, *Journal of Wound Care*, Volume 3, Issue 2, pp. 198–201, Copyright © 2013 HMP Communications; and Cutting CF and White R., Defined and refined: Criteria for identifying wound infection revisited, *British Journal of Community Nursing*, Volume 9, Issue 3, pp. S6–15, Copyright © 2004 MA Healthcare Limited.

A position document has been produced by the European Wound Management Association to further consolidate criteria for infection (European Wound Management Association, 2005).

What is specific immunity?

The specific immune response is a series of adaptive changes, triggered in response to individual organisms or components of microorganisms, resulting in the production of specific antibodies. These are activated due to the recognition of specific antigens produced by or present on the surface of the pathogen. In the early response (or primary response), immunoglobulin IgM is produced, which is then replaced by large amounts of IgG (secondary response). In mucous membranes, IgA is produced in abundance. These specific antibodies will protect from future infection and inactivate the pathogen and prepare it for destruction.

Whilst there have been huge advances in understanding the immune system and the wound healing process, the interaction of microorganism in this process is sometimes overlooked.

 KEY POINT

Antigens are made from amino acids or sugar residues linked together to form short sequences. The short sequences are termed epitopes and can be derived from toxins, surface proteins on virus-infected cells.

Conclusion

In the United Kingdom, there is estimated to be over 300,000 patients at any one time living with chronic wounds causing problems to their general day-to-day living and impeding their quality of life (Posnett and Franks 2008). The true cost to an individual cannot be estimated, although there is a monetary value placed on the healthcare costs. Why an individual with no evident impediment to their immune system develops a non-healing wound is confounding numerous wound care practitioners. In many cases, no matter what treatment strategy is applied to the wound, the normal wound healing process appears to be halted in the inflammatory phase. Whether this is due to overproduction of host factors such as matrix metalloproteases, or a wound biofilm, or both, affecting the immune response and wound healing process needs further investigation. New technologies are in development to try to answer some of these questions but until they are available and have been adequately tested, then as practitioners unfortunately you must continue to address problem wounds empirically and perhaps assume the interaction of microorganisms and/or products they produce, are impeding the wound healing process.

Further reading

Ford M. *Medical Microbiology* (2nd ed). Oxford: Oxford University Press; 2014.

Goering RV, Dockrell H, Zuckerman M, *et al. Mims Medical Microbiology* (7th ed). Philadelphia, PA: Saunders; 2013.

References

Cooke J. Infectious diseases – the need for new antibiotics. *Hosp Pharm.* 2004;**11**: 265–268.

Cutting KF, Harding KG. Criteria for identifying wound infection. *J Wound Care.* 1994;**3**(4):198–201.

Cutting CF, White R. Defined and refined: criteria for identifying wound infection revisited. *Br J Community Nurs.* 2004;**9**(3):S6–15.

Elliott IMZ. *A Short History of Surgical Dressings.* London: The Pharmaceutical Press; 1964.

European Wound Management Association. *Identifying Criteria for Wound Infection.* Position document. London: MEP Ltd; 2005.

Forrest RD. Early history of wound treatment. *J Royal Soc Med.* 1982;**75**:198–205.

Posnett J, Franks PJ. The burden of chronic wounds in the UK. *Nurs Times.* 2008;**104**(3):44–45.

Chapter 2

Microbiology: the basics

Valerie Edwards-Jones

Objectives

This chapter covers the structure and taxonomy of microorganisms and describes important differences between them. On completing this chapter you should have knowledge and understanding of:

1 The structure of all major groups of microorganisms
2 The difference between prokaryotic and eukaryotic cells
3 How to distinguish between bacteria, viruses, fungi, and parasites
4 The growth of bacteria and be able to outline the infectious process
5 The importance of each in human disease with specific examples for the wound care professional.

Introduction to the basics of microbiology

The higher forms of animals and plants are very complex structures of different cell types with different functions and can be seen by the naked eye. Microorganisms on the other hand are **usually** single-celled and visualized under a microscope. There is as much diversity in the microscopic world as the world that can be seen by the naked eye. We therefore use a range of characteristics to help with diagnosis of infectious disease. These include clinical features of the illness, detection of the organisms in the clinical sample, microscopic appearance, and growth characteristics. Identification of the organism and how it behaves in the environment and the human body is important so that we can monitor how disease patterns change so as to hopefully prevent future occurrence. The process of determining the pattern of disease development is termed epidemiology and it is essential for this process that everyone in healthcare understands some basic features of microbiology and infectious disease.

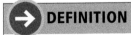

DEFINITION

Epidemiology is the study of patterns, causes, and effects of health and disease conditions in populations.

One key area that will help wound care practitioners successfully manage infected wounds is understanding the differences between the major groups of microorganisms, how they are classified, and named, so that the correct treatment can be administered and epidemiological information maintained.

There are four major groups of microorganisms:

- Bacteria
- Fungi (including yeast)
- Parasites
- Viruses.

These groups can be further subdivided and there are thousands of microorganisms within each group. The system of organizing or classifying these microorganisms is known as **microbial taxonomy**. Structure (anatomy) and function (processes, metabolism, etc.) of the microorganism is very important and frequently used in classification. The microorganisms are formally assigned names that are recognized across the world and this allows accurate communication about infectious disease to be relayed. The system of naming a microorganism (nomenclature) most commonly used in microbiology is the Linnaean scheme (after a Swedish botanist Carl von Linné), which is based on the common language of Latin. The basic scheme divides the living world into seven different subdivisions: **kingdom, phylum, class, order, family, genus**, and **species**. The two most commonly used divisions in microbiology are the genus name (e.g. *Staphylococcus*) and the species name (e.g. *aureus*), as in *Staphylococcus aureus*.

DEFINITION

- **Microbial taxonomy** is the process of organizing or classifying organisms into different groups and subgroups.
- **Nomenclature** is the system of naming a microorganism.

FACT

The taxonomic rank **kingdom** is divided into five different subdivisions: **Animalia** (vertebrates and invertebrates), **Plantae** (plants), **Fungi, Protista,** and **Monera** (containing eubacteria).

KEY POINT

The scientific name assigned to a microorganism consists of **genus** and **species**, written in italics or underlined, with the first letter of the genus in upper case and the species in lower case, for example, *Staphylococcus aureus.*

There have been changes to some organism names over the last few decades as more accurate methods have been used to confirm their identity and assign them to the correct genus. This can be very confusing for the healthcare professional when the different names are being used in everyday practice. For example, group A strep is a common name used for the bacterium, *Streptococcus pyogenes.*

KEY POINT

For example: the causative organism of scarlet fever is *Streptococcus pyogenes* but this is known by several other names:
- *Streptococcus pyogenes* (genus and species name)
- *S. pyogenes* (proper abbreviated name)
- *Strep. pyogenes* (colloquial name)
- Streptococci (group name)
- Group A strep (common name).

Different groups of microorganisms

Bacteria

Bacteria are single-celled organisms known as prokaryotes which have important differences from eukaryotes that facilitate their survival and treatment. Table 2.1 highlights the differences between a prokaryotic and eukaryotic cell.

Table 2.1 The major differences between a eukaryote cell (human cell) and a prokaryote cell (bacterial cell)

	Prokaryote	Eukaryote
Nuclear structure and processes		
Nuclear membrane	Absent	Present
Chromosomes	Single chromosome (haploid)	Pairs of chromosomes (diploid)
Nuclear division	No mitosis	Mitosis
Cytoplasm structures and processes		
Ribosome	70s	80s
Mitochondria, Golgi apparatus, endoplasmic reticulum	Absent	Present
Cell wall (peptidoglycan)	Present	Absent

Bacteria possess both deoxyribonucleic acid (DNA) and ribonucleic acid (RNA). They have no defined nucleus, mitochondria or other organelles enclosed in a membrane, which means that any structure is free floating in the cytoplasm. They usually have a rigid **cell wall** (there are exceptions, e.g. *Mycoplasma*) consisting of a polymer of amino sugars, *N*-acetyl muramic acid, and *N*-acetyl glucosamine called peptidoglycan. This structure is not seen in eukaryotic cells which make it an ideal target for some antimicrobial compounds (e.g. penicillins and cephalosporins).

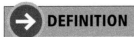 **DEFINITION**

Peptidoglycan is a polymer of two amino sugars and is unique to bacteria. It is the target site for penicillin.

The outer layer of the cell wall can vary between different bacterial species but may include structures such as **pili, fimbriae,** and **flagella.** Some species have a **capsule**, usually polysaccharide, which is external to the cell wall and is a common pathogenic mechanism which helps the bacteria resist phagocytosis by macrophages, and also helps with adhesion to tissue cells. The basic bacterial structure is diagrammatically represented in Figure 2.1 and the individual structures described in Table 2.2.

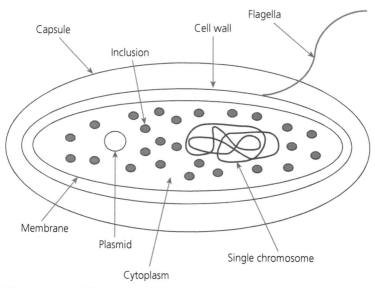

Figure 2.1 The different structures found on a bacterial cell.

Table 2.2 Major structures of a bacterial cell

Pili and fimbriae	Hair-like structures that stick out from the cell surface of some species. They help with adhesion and consist mainly of protein
Flagella	Long, thin structures that are responsible for movement. Bacteria can have a single flagellum or multiple flagella at different parts of the cell
Spores	These form a very dense protective coat that helps the bacterial cell resist adverse conditions. Commonly seen in *Bacillus* spp. or *Clostridia* spp. Helpful with identification of the organism

(Continued)

Table 2.2 (continued) Major structures of a bacterial cell

DNA	Bacterial DNA is a single, supercoiled chromosome. It is *not* surrounded by a nuclear membrane. There may also be plasmids inside a bacterial cell. These are extrachromosomal DNA
Cell envelope	Consists of outer membrane, cell wall, and cytoplasmic membrane
Outer membrane	Only found in Gram-negative bacteria, consists of lipopolysaccharide
Cell wall	Rigid polymer consisting of alternating groups of *N*-acetylmuramic acid and *N*-acetylglucosamine, which forms peptidoglycan. Of varying thickness, with Gram-positive organisms having a thicker cell wall than Gram-negative organisms
Cell membrane	Cell membrane consists of lipid bilayer and enclosed by a thick cell wall (exception: *Mycoplasma* spp. do not have a cell wall)
Capsule	External to cell wall but still attached to the bacteria. Most commonly consists of polysaccharide but odd exceptions (*Bacillus anthracis*) can have a protein capsule
Slime layer (glycocalyx)	External to the cell wall but often secreted and not firmly attached. Consists mainly of polysaccharide

How do we assign bacteria into their species?

Bacteria are divided into general groups based on the staining reaction and biochemical tests used frequently in the laboratory (e.g. microscopic shape and Gram reaction), nutritional and biochemical requirements (e.g. requirement for oxygen, temperature dependence, pH, and lactose utilization production of catalase enzyme), immunological status (e.g. antigens present on their surface), and more recently using genetic and protein markers (e.g. gene sequencing, presence of specific genes, and protein patterns).

In addition to helping assign bacteria to particular taxa, understanding their physiology, structure, biochemistry, and nutritional status also allows the microbiologist to understand their pathogenicity (ability to cause disease) and possible treatment.

Other biochemical and genetic techniques are used to identify bacteria fully and some of the traditional methods will be described further in Chapter 3.

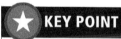

KEY POINT

The Gram stain is the most important staining process used in diagnostic microbiology and was named after the Danish bacteriologist Hans Christian Gram who published this method in 1884. It is a simple procedure and distinguishes between two classes of bacteria, **Gram-positive** and **Gram-negative** bacteria. It makes use of a primary stain (crystal violet) which complexes with the cell wall in Gram-positive bacteria and stains them purple, and a secondary stain (safranin) which counterstains the other bacteria red, where the complex is not formed (Gram-negative). Examples of Gram-positive and Gram-negative bacteria are shown in Figure 2.2.

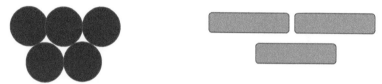

Figure 2.2 Gram-positive (left) and Gram-negative (right) bacteria.

Other staining methods are available that show the presence of other bacterial structures such as granules, capsules, flagella, and spores. Also other sophisticated staining methods can help with identification (e.g. auramine/phenol stain for tuberculosis in sputum, using a fluorescent stain).

The shape of the bacterial cell determined by microscopy is also used in identification and is important in taxonomy. There are four fundamental shapes: spherical, rod-shaped, spiral, and comma-shaped, represented in Figure 2.3.

- Coccus (spherical)
- Bacillus (rod-shaped)
- Spirochaetes (spiral rods)   1 μm
- Curved rods (comma-shaped)

Figure 2.3 Bacterial shapes.

KEY POINT

Examples of the medically important bacteria demonstrated by Gram stain and found in wound care are:

- Gram-positive cocci:
  Staphylococcus aureus
  Streptococcus pyogenes
- Gram-positive bacilli:
  Clostridium perfringens (gas gangrene)
- Gram-negative bacilli:
  Pseudomonas aeruginosa
  Escherichia coli.

Viruses

Viruses are extremely small and can only be seen using electron microscopy that magnifies up to 10,000 times. They contain either RNA or DNA usually in linear form and they have a coat of protein subunits (**capsomeres**) which together form a nucleocapsid. In some species, there may also be a lipid envelope. They may show structural similarities such as a helical or icosahedral symmetry or have no particular symmetry at all. They are obligate intracellular parasites and as such can only grow and proliferate within living cells. They are host specific (e.g. bacteriophages are viruses that attack bacteria, animal viruses only attack animals, human viruses only attack humans). Viruses are named according to the disease they are responsible for, and the taxonomic system is not the same as for bacteria. Figure 2.4 shows a diagram of a single-stranded RNA-enveloped virus (human immunodeficiency virus) with the various external features which help with attachment and virulence of the virus.

→ DEFINITION

- **Nucleocapsid** is a protein coat that forms the outer surface of virus and contains the nucleic acid.
- **Obligate intracellular parasites** are parasites that, by necessity, live inside cells.

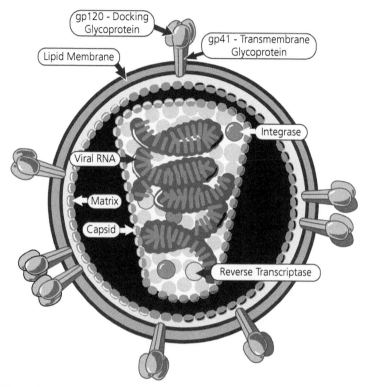

Figure 2.4 Diagram of the human immunodeficiency virus (HIV).

Reproduced from Centers for Disease Control and Prevention, Public Health Image Library (PHIL), Image ID# 18163, National Institute of Allergy and Infectious Diseases (NIAID), 2010, available from http://phil.cdc.gov/phil/details.asp?pid=18163.

There are two main classes of viruses—DNA viruses and RNA viruses—that can be further subclassified depending upon whether they are single stranded or double stranded.

For example:

- **Single-stranded DNA viruses** include parvoviruses (parvovirus B19 responsible for Fifth's disease, also known as slapped cheek syndrome)
- **Double-stranded DNA viruses** include pox viruses (responsible for smallpox) and herpes viruses (responsible for herpes simplex, genital herpes, or cold sores)

◆ **Single-stranded RNA viruses** include orthomyxovirus (responsible for influenza) and retroviruses (responsible for acquired immunodeficiency syndrome (AIDS)).

Viruses can cause a number of human diseases, which involve the skin. A common problem is the production of vesicles (e.g. with chicken pox and small pox).

Fungi

Fungi are eukaryotes containing both RNA and DNA. They have a defined nucleus and a complex cell wall containing sterols (which are the target sites of many antifungal agents), chitin, glucans, mannans, and glycoproteins. All fungi can reproduce sexually (telemorphic state) and asexually (anamorphic state). Sometimes the fungi can be given different names depending upon how they are referred to. Infections in humans are collectively called 'mycoses' and skin infections commonly termed tinea infections.

 KEY POINT

There are two major morphologic forms of fungi:

1 **Yeasts** (small round unicellular fungi), for example, *Candida* spp. (see Figure 2.5)

2 **Moulds** (grow as filamentous forms), for example, *Penicillium* spp. (see Figure 2.6).

A third type, **dimorphic fungi,** can exist in both forms with the yeast form existing in the body at higher temperatures and the filamentous form in the environment at lower temperatures. An example of the disease caused by this type of fungus is *Histoplasma capsulatum*.

Usually fungal infections are described based on the clinical disease they cause:

◆ **Superficial mycoses:** fungal infection commonly infecting the epidermis of skin (e.g. tinea versicolor)

◆ **Cutaneous mycoses:** dermatophyte (skin-loving) infections (e.g. ringworm and *Trichophyton rubrum*)

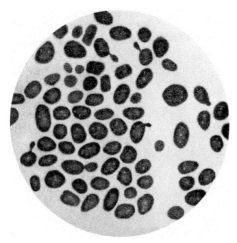

Figure 2.5 Microscopic image of yeast cells (note some have buds on the oval cells which is diagnostic).

Reproduced from Centers for Disease Control and Prevention, Public Health Image Library (PHIL), Image ID# 14353, CDC, 1979, available from http://phil.cdc.gov/phil/details. asp?pid=14353.

- ◆ **Subcutaneous mycoses**: chronic localized infections of the skin and subcutaneous tissue usually following implantation of the fungal agent during trauma, termed mycetoma (e.g. *Sporothrix schenckii*)
- ◆ **Systemic/deep mycoses**: originate in the lungs and spread through the body, for example, *Histoplasmosis*. These are usually dimorphic fungi and often found in people with immune deficiencies, for example, patients with cancer or AIDs.

Most wound care practitioners will come across superficial yeast infections in chronic wounds. They are easy to isolate and identify from a wound and the commonest yeast is *Candida albicans*. Most yeasts respond to topical antiseptics but if they begin to invade then systemic antifungal agents may need to be prescribed. Dermatophyte infections are often seen in dermatology, and skin scrapings, hair, or nail clippings are taken for diagnosis in the laboratory. Both microscopy and culture are used to identify fungal infections. Dermatophytes are grown and identified in the laboratory but they grow much more slowly than bacteria and isolation and identification can take approximately 3 weeks. They are treated with an antifungal agent

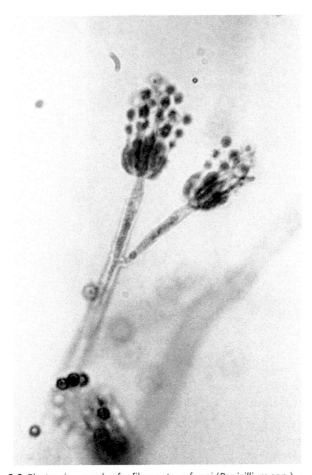

Figure 2.6 Photomicrograph of a filamentous fungi (*Penicillium* spp.).

Reproduced from Centers for Disease Control and Prevention, Public Health Image Library (PHIL), Image ID# 8398, Lucille Georg, available from http://phil.cdc.gov/phil/details. asp?pid=8398.

(terbinafine). The commonest dermatophyte infection is athlete's foot (tinea pedis), most frequently caused by *Trichophyton rubrum*. The fungus grows relatively quickly (approximately 1 week) on dermatophyte culture media and is identified by the hyphae and the colour of the colony when grown. An example is shown in Figure 2.7.

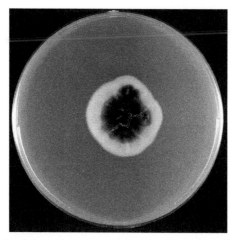

Figure 2.7 *Trichophyton rubrum* growing on dermatophyte culture medium. The underside of the colony is a reddy brown colour and the upper side of the colony is often white.

Parasites

Parasites are eukaryotes and cause a range of diseases in humans. Parasites can be single-celled (e.g. protozoa), which will necessitate diagnosis based on the microscopic structures of their cells, eggs, or ova. Parasites can also be multicellular organisms such as worms, and can be visible by the naked eye. They all have complex life cycles and are usually identified in the laboratory by their morphology. Parasites are divided into a number of different subdivisions based on their morphology and disease manifestation. Very basically, parasites are classified as single-celled protozoa (sporazoa and flagellates) and multicelled helminths (cestodes, nematodes, and trematodes). Examples of the common parasites in each group are shown in Table 2.3. In wound care, ectoparasites may cause a wound following a bite (e.g. scabies) and very rarely, humans may become an alternative host and a fly may unintentionally lay their eggs under the skin causing an abnormal wound and swelling (as seen with blow fly larva).

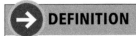

> **DEFINITION**
>
> An **ectoparasite** is a parasite that lives on the skin or body but not within the body.

Parasites are rarely encountered as a cause of chronic wounds, but can cause an acute wound (following a tick bite) which can progress to create a chronic wound if left untreated or inappropriately treated. An excellent example of this is Lyme disease, where a spirochaete bacterium, *Borrelia burgdorferi*, is injected into the skin following a tick bite (usually by an *Ixodes* spp. tick). A typical itchy localized 'bull's eye' lesion (erythema chronicum migrans) is formed which responds very well to antibiotics (penicillins). If left untreated the spirochaete can disseminate causing further complications to the nervous system, joints, and heart.

Examples of some common human parasites are shown in Table 2.3.

Table 2.3 Brief outline of common human parasitic diseases

Protozoa (single-celled)	
Sporozoa:	*Plasmodium* spp. (malaria)
Flagellates:	Intestinal, e.g. *Trichomonas vaginalis*
	Blood, e.g. *Leishmania* spp.
Helminths (worms)	
Cestodes:	Flatworms, tapeworms
Nematodes:	Roundworms, e.g. *Ascaris* spp.
Trematodes:	Flukes, e.g. schistosomiasis (bilharzia)

Growth and reproduction of bacteria

The most frequently encountered microorganisms in wounds (both acute and chronic) are bacteria. Therefore, their growth and role in the infectious process will be described in more detail within this chapter. Further information on viruses, fungi, and parasites is available in the books listed in 'Further reading'.

Bacteria reproduce using asexual reproduction or binary fission and produce identical daughter cells, unless there is some mutational event. Growth in the laboratory (*in vitro*) is quite different to growth in a patient (*in vivo*) and this can be difficult to model because of the effects of the immune system.

Bacterial growth in the laboratory

When a single bacterial cell is placed into new growth medium in the laboratory and is given ideal conditions to grow (nutrients, temperature, oxygen requirements, etc.), it follows a typical pattern (called the **growth curve**) using four **phases** of growth (**lag, log, stationary,** and **decline** phases) (see Figure 2.8). In the laboratory there are no barriers to growth (such as the immune system in the human body) and the bacteria will continue to grow until the nutrients expire or toxic products build up. They will then die unless the bacterium utilizes some mechanism for survival. A common survival mechanism used by some bacterial species is the production of spores and these are produced by common bacteria such as *Clostridium* spp. and *Bacillus* spp. Spores have a number of features, they can tolerate extreme dryness, some cannot be killed at high or low temperatures, and some are resistant to antiseptics and disinfectants.

During the **lag** phase, the organism is adapting to its new environment and it is usually during this stage that adhesions are produced to allow the organism to attach to any surfaces. This will be highly dependent upon the physical material and structure of the surface. Following adaptation, the organism enters the **logarithmic** (log) or **exponential** phase where it begins to grow by binary fission. The bacterial cells double at regular intervals (**doubling time**). This time period can be as low as 20 minutes in the laboratory. Therefore within a number of hours (approximately 6 hours), a single bacterial cell can increase in numbers from 1 cell to 1 million cells (10^6 cells). During the log phase the bacterial cells are under strict regulatory control based on nutrient availability and the cells produce autoregulatory molecules (signalling molecules) which accumulate in the growth medium. These enable a single cell to sense the number of bacteria in the growth medium and this communication between cells is known as quorum sensing (Williams et al. 2007). This biological communication allows the bacteria to coordinate their behaviour and is used in the production of toxins for invasion, production of spores for survival, or production of biofilms (Cotter and Miller 1998). These molecules have been identified in many species and are N-acyl-homoserine lactone (HSL) molecules in Gram-negative bacteria and an octapeptide in Gram-positive bacteria (Ji et al. 1995).

Once the nutrients become depleted, the bacteria grow and die at the same rate, resulting in a stabilization of organism numbers (**stationary** phase), and eventually the numbers dying outnumber those growing and the organism enters the **decline** phase.

Having some knowledge of the four phases of bacterial growth helps to understand how some bacteria either colonize or infect a wound depending on their growth conditions and survival mechanisms and whether they invade the tissue or form a biofilm as part of a survival mode of growth. In addition, it can help explain why organism numbers, production of toxins, and quorum sensing have such important roles to play in the differentiation between colonization and infection. Reduction in the levels of communication molecules and bacterial numbers through exudate management, cleansing, and debridement should help reduce inhibition of growth factors by the extracellular toxins and enzymes produced by the bacteria.

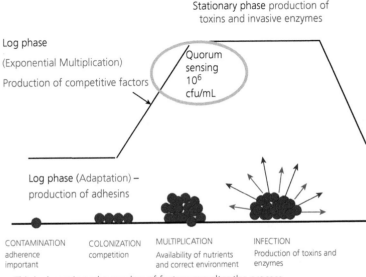

Figure 2.8 Typical bacterial growth curve in batch culture (i.e. bacteria placed in a nutritionally supportive growth medium and allowed to grow uninterrupted in optimum growth conditions). The infectious process (depicted as contamination, colonization, multiplication, and infection) is represented below the growth curve at the respective stages.

How does a microorganism cause wound infection?

Most wound infections are caused by bacteria, although very occasionally, viruses or fungi can be implicated. A successful pathogen must overcome the host innate defences and although each pathogen will have its own specific mechanism of causing infection, in general the infectious process is the same (Edwards-Jones 2010).

★ KEY POINT

Infection process

The general infection process occurs in four stages: **attachment, colonization, multiplication,** and **invasion.**

In order for a microorganism to cause active infection, the host defence mechanisms have to be overcome and the microorganism invades the tissues. The microorganism can remain at the site of entry (local infection) or eventually become disseminated throughout the body (systemic infection). Dissemination is common with many viral infections but most bacterial, parasitic, and fungal infections remain localized.

Some pathogens can penetrate the skin once it is broken through trauma, bites, burns, or surgery. Occasionally some pathogens can cause skin infection by penetrating the hair shaft, usually through production of toxins. Most breaks in the skin become colonized with microorganisms very rapidly and whether or not an infection develops depends upon the virulence of the organism and the susceptibility of the host.

! FACT

Virulence can be quantified by the LD_{50} (lethal dose 50)—the lowest inoculum required to kill 50% of experimental animals

Most microorganisms (bacteria, fungi, and parasites) follow a typical infection pathway (**attachment, colonization, multiplication,** and **invasion**) but viral infection varies slightly with specific attachment and internalization occurring within 30 minutes, followed by multiplication and release (which results in the destruction of the host cell). Viral infection is hugely efficient and results in a huge expansion in the number of viral particles.

The common infection pathway follows:

- Tissue will be contaminated by a potential microorganism and attachment to the tissue will follow. **Attachment** is dependent upon the microorganism and can be a specific or non-specific reaction.
- **Non-specific attachment** is often reversible and examples include chemical hydrophobic/hydrophilic reactions and interactive forces

between the surface of the microbe and the host. The environment greatly influences this process and the presence of adhesins is under the control of genetic regulation mechanisms of the microbe.

- ◆ **Specific adherence** involves irreversible formation of bonds between complementary molecules on each cell surface and is known as the ligand–receptor reaction. Enzymes and chemicals can inhibit this reaction and the host can also produce protective antibodies that will inhibit attachment.

 KEY POINT

A ligand receptor is a binding site on the host surface that various adhesion molecules attach to.

Adhesion or attachment is the most important stage of the infection process and a variety of surface-associated components are involved (Table 2.4). Common wound pathogens such as *Staphylococcus aureus, Pseudomonas aeruginosa*, and *Streptococcus pyogenes* each have their own virulence factors to allow attachment. *S. aureus* produce surface proteins that bind to collagen, fibronectin, and fibrinogen (Foster and Hook 1998). *P. aeruginosa* attach by a secreted polysaccharide, alginate, which is also used in the formation of stable biofilms (these are discussed in detail in Chapter 6).

Colonization is the next stage of infection and is highly dependent upon the ability of the microorganism to evade the immune cells (macrophages and neutrophils) and cytokines released during the inflammatory response. Some microorganisms produce molecules which interfere with phagocytosis and chemotaxis. Attachment and colonization represent the lag phase in the laboratory bacterial growth cycle.

 DEFINITION

Chemotaxis is the movement of a phagocyte in response to a chemical stimulation or cytokine.

Multiplication is the next stage of the infection process. The microorganisms divide rapidly utilizing all the available nutrients, and secrete toxins to aid invasion, the final stage of the infection process. During this stage the

Table 2.4 A list of commonly used terms to describe adherence factors

Adherence factor	Description of mechanism	Microorganism using this mechanism to adhere to the host
Adhesin	A surface structure that enables a bacterial cell to attach to a host cell	
Lectin	A protein structure that binds to carbohydrate on the host tissue	
Ligand	A surface molecule that binds specifically to a receptor molecule on another surface	
Receptor	A binding site on the host surface that binds ligands or adhesins	
Capsule	A layer of polysaccharide on the surface of a bacterial cell	*Klebsiella pneumoniae*
Slime layer	Proteins secreted from microbial cells	*Staphylococcus epidermidis*
Teichoic acids and lipoteichoic acids (LTAs)	Cell wall components of Gram-positive bacteria	*Staphylococcus aureus*
Fimbriae	Filamentous proteins on the surface of bacterial cells	Type 1 fimbriae of *Escherichia coli*
Lipopolysaccharide (LPS)	A cell wall component of the outer membrane of Gram-negative bacteria	*Escherichia coli*

amount of exudate will begin to increase and odour will start developing. This is represented by the log or exponential phase in the laboratory bacterial growth cycle.

Invasion is the final stage of the infection process and the microorganism will invade deeper tissues to release a further supply of nutrients. This is under regulated control by quorum sensing molecules and represents the late exponential phase of the laboratory bacterial growth cycle. Many pathogens produce an array of toxins or enzymes that can kill phagocytic cells, destroy cell membranes, inhibit complement, and cause metabolic imbalance of the cell. It is during this stage that clinical signs of infection become visible.

The first signs are redness, swelling, pain, and heat. Other symptoms may follow, including production of pus as the cells break down. Necrosis can result leading to massive tissue destruction.

 FACT

Process of pathogen recognition

The phagocyte recognizes the pathogen as foreign and engulfs it. Inside the phagocyte the pathogen is exposed to a variety of chemicals (hydrogen peroxide and oxygen radicals) and enzymes (lactoperoxidase) and is digested. The antigens released from the digested organisms are pushed through the membrane of the phagocyte and are 'presented' to circulating lymphocytes (B cells and T cells) of the immune system, which activates the specific immune system and antibodies and cytokines (chemicals produced by cells) are produced to further activate both the non-specific and specific immune system.

Conclusion

Bacteria, viruses, fungi, and parasites can cause a range of infectious disease in humans and the clinical presentation of the disease varies depending upon the individual (primarily due to differences between immune systems) and the virulence factors produced by the microorganism. Only certain microorganisms will cause skin and soft tissue infection, including acute and chronic wounds. Recent research has shown that chronic wounds are the result of the formation of biofilms on the surface of the wound and chronicity may remain *ad infinitum* unless there is some external disruption to the biofilm. Newer techniques are being made available to the microbiologist, and with collaboration with the wound care specialist, these techniques are helping to explain some of the complex interactions that occur between the microorganism and the wound bed during the wound healing process. As this becomes better understood, there will be an excellent opportunity for new wound care products to be produced.

Further reading

Carroll KC, Brooks GF, Butel JS, *et al. Jawetz, Melnick & Adelberg's Medical Microbiology* (26th ed). New York: Lange Medical Books, McGraw Hill Education; 2013.

Ford M. *Medical Microbiology* (2nd ed). Oxford: Oxford University Press; 2014.

Goering RV, Dockrell H, Zuckerman M, *et al. Mims Medical Microbiology* (7th ed). Philadelphia, PA: Saunders; 2013.

Murray PR, Rosenthal KS, Pfaller MA. *Medical Microbiology* (7th ed). Orlando, FL: Mosby Inc; 2013.

Todar K. *Todar's Online Textbook of Bacteriology.* Department of Bacteriology, University of Wisconsin. Available from: http://www.textbookofbacteriology.net/

References

Cotter PA, Millet JF. *In vivo* and *ex vivo* regulation of bacterial virulence gene expression. *Curr Opin Microbiol.* 1998;1:17–26.

Edwards-Jones V. The science of infection. *Wounds UK.* 2010;6(2):86–93.

Foster TJ, Hook M. Surface protein adhesins of Staphylococcus aureus. *Trends Microbiol.* 1998;6:484–488.

Ji G, Beavls RC, Novick RP. Cell density control of staphylococcal virulence mediated by an octapeptide pheromone. *Proc Natl Acad Sci U S A.* 1995;92:12055–12059.

Williams P, Winzer K, Chan WC, *et al.* Look who's talking: communication and quorum sensing in the bacterial world Phil. *Trans R Soc B.* 2007;362:1119–1134.

Chapter 3

Collection, transport, and laboratory processing of wound, tissue, and bone samples

Geoff Edwards-Jones

Objectives

This chapter describes the laboratory diagnosis of infection with specific reference to wound infection. On completing this chapter you should have knowledge and understanding of:

1 Procedures used in sample collection
2 Sample types and their collection used in laboratory diagnosis of wound infection
3 The importance of sample transport and regulations associated with them
4 The variety of methods used during sample processing
5 Identification of microorganisms
6 Health and safety considerations.

Introduction to infected wound sample collection and processing

A clean, non-infected acute wound will usually heal normally even if there is slight contamination with normal skin organisms. However a dirty, chronic, or large wound may become heavily colonized with microorganisms, which may or may not then lead to infection. In the majority of cases, these infecting organisms are bacteria, although in some (rare) cases, viruses or fungi may be implicated. The current chapter restricts itself to the diagnosis of bacterial wound infections, which cause the majority of problems in both acute and chronic wounds.

Diagnosis of wound infection

The diagnosis of wound infection depends on both clinical and microbiological assessment, the latter being both complex and time-consuming. For accurate microbiological diagnosis, the quality of the **sample** (or specimen) taken from the wound and the detailed information supplied on the specimen request form is very important. Details such as antibiotic usage, foreign travel (in case of rare pathogens), cause of trauma (dog bites, human bites, etc.), age, sex, and other medical conditions must be noted. All laboratory assessments and results will be dependent on these. Subsequent storage, transport, and laboratory processing of the sample are also crucial to an accurate microbiological diagnosis.

Sample collection

In general, all clinical samples should be collected before the patient is given any antibiotics, so that recovery of bacteria from the sample is not compromised. This is particularly true of samples from sterile sites such as blood cultures and urine, but also applies to collection of wound samples. For example, the patient may be on long-term antibiotics for a chest or urinary tract infection, and this may compromise the isolation of potential pathogens from the wound. Therefore, it is important that the laboratory is informed of the patient's current antibiotic treatment as the laboratory may process the sample in a different manner.

 KEY POINT

Sample collection

◆ **Provide sufficient sample**: culture of wound material in the laboratory is often complex and may involve several different procedures for diagnosis including culture and microscopy, hence sufficient material must be provided to accommodate this. If pus is present, aspirate as much as possible with a sterile syringe and needle and place in a sterile container before transporting to the laboratory.

◆ **Use appropriate containers**: all sterile swabs and containers are provided by the processing laboratory. Do not use non-sterile containers.

KEY POINT (continued)

- **Correct labelling**: all microbiological samples must be correctly labelled with appropriate patient details. If more than one sample is taken from a large wound, then each sample site should be identified accordingly (e.g. external surface, wound floor, etc.). All samples must be accompanied by a request form which must contain sufficient information to correctly identify the patient (full patient name, date of birth, and hospital or NHS number). In addition, the request form should include as much clinical information as possible that is relevant to the investigations required. For example, site of wound, nature of the wound (e.g. surgical or penetrating injury), any underlying pathology (e.g. diabetes), current antibiotic therapy (give antibiotic names), and any topical treatment being administered.

 FACT

One of the commonest reasons for laboratories not processing samples is insufficient and/or inaccurate completion of the request form and/or sample container.

When collecting any sample for laboratory processing, care must be taken to avoid contamination with extraneous bacteria, for example, from the area surrounding the wound, from the healthcare worker collecting the sample, or from non-sterile equipment. This is achieved by using strict **aseptic technique**. Patient compliance should be sought and an explanation given as to the nature and reason for the procedures to be used.

 KEY POINT

Aseptic technique is a procedure performed under sterile conditions. This is undertaken during sample collection using sterile equipment and ensuring good hygiene practices. This general good practice should protect the health worker from potential infection.

Sampling the wound

Wound infection occurs within viable wound tissue, not in necrotic tissue or other debris associated with wounds; therefore prior to taking a sample, the wound must be cleansed (using sterile saline, water, or antimicrobial washes) to remove unattached microorganisms. Also, any necrotic tissue or eschar (scab) should be removed before sampling.

If the wound is washed with an antimicrobial wash or has been previously dressed with an antimicrobial dressing, it is important that any residual antimicrobial substances should be rinsed away before sampling as they may affect the recovery of certain species of bacteria.

 KEY POINT

A wound must be thoroughly cleansed and any necrotic tissue debrided prior to sampling as microorganisms causing infection will be present in the wound bed. Any residual antimicrobial substance from dressings or washes must be rinsed away before sampling as this may affect the recovery of certain species of bacteria.

Sample types

Wound swab

A number of different types of swab are available and are supplied sterile. They consist of a holder, a shaft (wooden, plastic, or metal), and a compact ball of cotton material at one end. The whole swab is contained in a protective plastic tube. The bottom end of the protective tube may contain **transport medium**, a semi-solid medium designed to maintain the viability of any bacteria on the swab during its transport to the laboratory. It is recommended that tubes containing transport medium always be used for collection of wound swabs. Figure 3.1 shows a variety of specimen containers used in microbiology.

 FACT

Although swabs are the most common wound specimen taken, there is no definitive evidence that they provide the best means of identifying bacterial wound infection. They only detect surface bacteria and generally can only sample a limited area. The survival of some bacteria on the swab during transportation is limited.

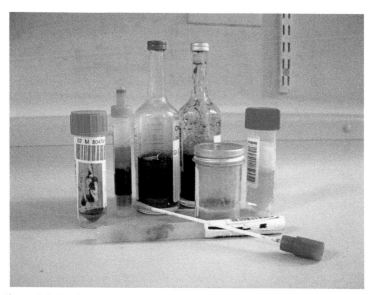

Figure 3.1 Specimen containers used in microbiology.

Taking a wound swab

If the wound is moist, then the swab can be used directly from the sterile packaging; however if the wound is dry, then the swab tip should be moistened with sterile saline. The most common method of taking a sample of the wound is the zig-zag sampling method, where the surface of the entire wound bed is swabbed in a zig-zag direction whilst simultaneously rotating the swab. Alternatively, the Levine technique (Levine et al. 1976) is used where the swab is rotated over a 1 cm square of tissue with sufficient pressure to express fluid from the tissue. It is considered that the Levine technique is probably more effective than the zig-zag procedure because it has the potential to release bacteria from within the tissue.

Biopsy

If a wound is long-standing or previous microbiological results have been inconclusive a biopsy sample from the wound may be useful. These samples often yield more accurate microbiological results as bacteria within the matrix of the tissue are isolated, rather than just surface bacteria. These samples are often taken during surgical interventions such as debridement of the wound.

The sample is taken aseptically with a scalpel or a punch biopsy instrument, which removes a plug of tissue (or bone). It is important to collect sufficient material to enable the laboratory to perform all the tests required, and the sample should be transferred to an appropriate laboratory container. These samples are accurately weighed and ground up in the laboratory using a tissue grinder (Griffiths tubes) prior to processing.

KEY POINT

Do not add formalin to any biopsy material for bacterial culture as it will kill any organisms present.

Pus

An infected wound usually generates pus and if there is sufficient available it should be aspirated using a sterile syringe and needle and transferred to an appropriate laboratory container.

A full description of these methods can be found elsewhere (Anonymous 2008).

Transport of specimens to the laboratory

After collecting the appropriate samples they should be transported to the processing laboratory as soon as possible because the bacteria contained in the samples may undergo various changes. Some bacteria such as staphylococci (e.g. *Staphylococcus aureus*) are fairly hardy and will be minimally affected; other species such as some anaerobic bacteria (e.g. *Bacteroides* spp.) will be acutely affected by the oxygen in the atmosphere and will begin to die immediately.

There are a number of consequences if transport is delayed:

♦ If there are small numbers of the infecting organism in the specimen then any depletion in numbers may make isolation of the organism more difficult, and in the worst case, isolation may be impossible.

♦ The relative numbers of bacteria within the sample may change. A fast-growing species may overgrow and give a false picture of numbers in the specimen. When there is more than one organism in the specimen, one species may outgrow another and inhibit growth of a more significant organism.

Storage of samples

If there is a delay in transporting wound samples to the laboratory, the samples should be stored until they can be collected. Swabs, particularly if they contain transport medium, should be stored at room temperature, away from sources of heat such as radiators. This will slow the rate of growth of most clinically significant bacteria and preserve relative bacterial numbers.

If a biopsy or other sample is obtained under anaesthetic, this should be processed as soon as possible. The laboratory should be contacted to discuss such samples and, if necessary, arrangements made for processing even outside normal laboratory hours.

Laboratory processing of wound samples

Microscopy

The laboratory may perform direct microscopic examination of the specimen (a Gram stain), to quickly assess the number and type of bacteria present in the sample. This is often useful for urgent samples where the clinician may wish to commence antibiotic therapy without delay, before culture results are available.

Culture

Traditionally, the main function of a microbiology laboratory is the isolation (or detection), and identification of all bacterial species in a given sample. In addition, the laboratory will perform antibiotic sensitivity tests on any pathogens isolated that are deemed to be significant. These traditional methods are time-consuming and time taken from receipt of specimen to a result being available is typically 24–48 hours.

Molecular methods, involving detection or expression of specific genes, have been introduced into some centres to help improve turnaround time, but currently these tests are only available for specific sample types and organisms. The most commonly used technique is the polymerase chain reaction (PCR) which will be described later in the chapter.

Microbiology laboratories process specimens based upon the nature of the sample (e.g. urine, sputum, and wound swabs) and the clinical information provided with the sample. The laboratory aims to isolate the most likely pathogens in a given sample by culturing the sample on a variety of culture media. Therefore a wound swab will always be cultured for the common pathogens (*Staphylococcus aureus* and *Pseudomonas* spp.); however, depending on specific clinical information provided, the laboratory may add additional culture media to look for rarer pathogens (e.g. *Pasteurella multocida* following a dog bite).

All procedures used in the laboratory for processing wound specimens use **aseptic techniques**, which are designed to maintain the integrity of the sample and avoid introducing extraneous bacteria into the sample or onto the culture plates. The wound swab or a portion of tissue or pus is physically applied to a segment of the surface of a selected culture plate by rubbing the samples over the agar surface, which allows the physical transfer of the bacteria from the sample to the surface of the plate. This is termed the main inoculum. The microbiologist, using a sterile bacteriological loop, will spread the deposited bacteria over the surface of the medium as shown in Figure 3.2. The purpose of spreading the inoculum is to separate the deposited bacteria so that after suitable incubation they will produce visible **bacterial colonies** as shown in Figure 3.3 and Figure 3.4.

 KEY POINT

The sample is rubbed onto the surface of a culture plate producing the main inoculum. A sterile loop is used to spread out the bacteria on the surface using a typical pattern shown in Figure 3.2. When the colonies only grow in the main inoculum, this is classed as a light or + growth; in the first spread, growth is classed as moderate or ++ growth; and if there is growth all across the plate it is classed as a heavy or +++ growth.

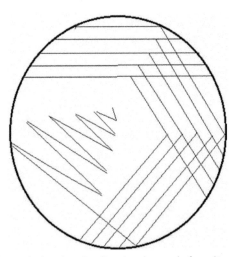

Figure 3.2 Schematic showing the directional spread of a culture plate.

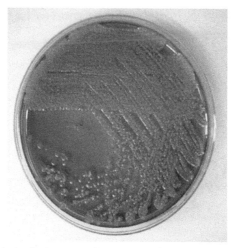

Figure 3.3 Typical colonies grown from a wound swab. This figure shows growth on CLED (cysteine lactose electrolyte deficient) media which is a general purpose media that allows growth of most common wound pathogens but inhibits the spreading effect of *Proteus* spp.

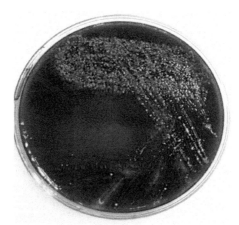

Figure 3.4 Typical colonies grown from a wound swab. This figure shows growth on Columbia blood agar, an enriched media (contains 5% horse blood) which has added nutrients. Note the *Proteus* spp. on Columbia agar spreading outwards from the colonies.

Environmental conditions required for bacterial growth

Temperature

Most clinically important bacteria can survive (and sometimes grow) over a wide temperature range (usually between 10°C and 60°C), but have an **optimum temperature** where growth is most rapid and luxuriant. This optimum temperature is usually 35–37°C.

Oxygen

The oxygen requirements of bacteria can be divided into the following three groups:

1 Aerobic bacteria—only grow in the presence of oxygen (e.g. *Pseudomonas aeruginosa*)

2 Anaerobic bacteria—only grow in the absence of oxygen (e.g. *Clostridium* spp.)

3 Facultative anaerobic bacteria—can grow in the presence or absence of oxygen (e.g. *Staphylococcus aureus*).

Laboratory incubators are set to provide the optimum temperature and there are specialized ones available to provide the correct gaseous requirements. Aerobic conditions are achieved by simply using the air, anaerobic conditions are achieved using sealed incubators with a piped gas supply (90% nitrogen, 5% carbon dioxide, and 5% hydrogen; see Figure 3.5) or small sealed containers (called anaerobic jars; see Figure 3.6), where the necessary gas mixture is generated using a disposable gas generating pack (e.g. GasPak™) (http://www.bd.com/ds/productCenter/ES-Gaspak.asp).

Facultative anaerobic bacteria

These bacteria can grow in the presence or absence of oxygen and will use a different metabolic pathway when oxygen is absent. This does have consequences on bacterial growth as they often grow more slowly and produce smaller colonies under anaerobic conditions. Many bacteria isolated from wound swabs are facultative anaerobes (such as *Staphylococcus* spp. and *Streptococcus* spp.).

 KEY POINT

It is important that the laboratory processing of any sample material from wounds includes incubation for both aerobic and anaerobic bacteria.

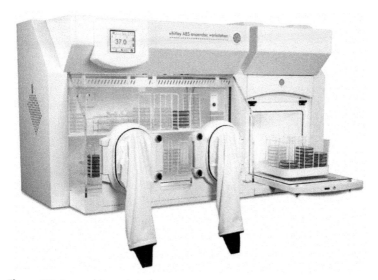

Figure 3.5 Anaerobic workstation.

Reproduced by kind permission of Don Whitley Scientific Ltd. Copyright © 2015 Don Whitley Scientific Ltd., UK.

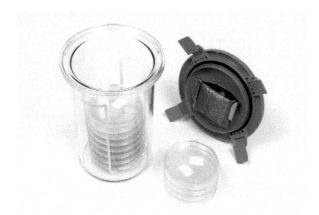

Figure 3.6 Anaerobic jar. The jar is assembled with a catalyst (in the lid) incubated in a normal incubator at 35–37°C. The atmosphere within the jar is free of oxygen, and consists mainly of nitrogen, with some carbon dioxide and hydrogen.

Reproduced by kind permission of Don Whitley Scientific Ltd. Copyright © 2015 Don Whitley Scientific Ltd., UK.

Nutrients

Essential nutrients are provided in microbiological culture media. There are two essential requirements of bacterial culture media:

1 The culture medium must contain all necessary chemical substances to support bacterial division and growth. These will include water, an energy source (glucose), a source of amino acids and other essential compounds for the production of proteins, nucleic acids, cell wall materials, and all other cellular components. These are supplied by substances called **peptones,** which are digests of animal and other proteins. In addition, an inert substance called **agar** (derived from various algae and seaweed) is added so that after the culture medium is sterilized at high temperature, the resulting material will solidify on cooling. The vast majority of bacterial culture media are in the form of a solid gel in petri dishes.

2 The final medium must be **sterile**, so that when a clinical sample is inoculated onto the culture medium, any bacteria growing on the medium are certain to have come from the sample alone, and not from any extraneous source.

Most modern culture media are supplied commercially in the form of dehydrated powder, which is reconstituted with the appropriate volume of distilled water. This suspension is then sterilized in an **autoclave,** at 121°C for 15 minutes. After appropriate cooling in a water bath at 50°C, the culture medium, still liquid, is dispensed into sterile plastic petri dishes in approximately 20 mL amounts to get the required depth in the petri dish. After cooling and setting, the culture medium (now colloquially called culture plates or agar plates) is allowed to dry overnight at room temperature. Finally, samples of the finished culture medium will undergo quality assurance before it is used to confirm the sterility of the medium and that it will grow the appropriate bacteria. Completed batches of medium are stored in a refrigerator for up to 3 weeks, until required for use.

Many laboratories purchase the culture media ready to use from commercial suppliers such as Oxoid, Lab M, and Difco. All media is supplied sterile, quality assured, and packaged ready for storage in a refrigerator.

A busy microbiology laboratory may use up to a dozen or more different culture media on a routine basis. In addition, there will be a number of more specialized media which are used only in certain circumstances (e.g. for the isolation of rare pathogens such as those that cause cholera or whooping cough). It is not uncommon for a large, busy microbiology laboratory to use several thousand agar plates a day.

In general, there are two main types of culture medium used in a micro-biology laboratory: **general purpose media** and **selective culture media**.

General purpose media

These contain all the essential requirements described in the previous section to enable the growth of most bacterial species. Material such as sterile blood (horse or sheep) may be added to improve the growth through addition of essential vitamins and minerals, required by more delicate organisms.

Selective culture media

This is a general purpose media with additives, such as chemicals, dyes, or antibiotics. These additional substances will promote the growth of certain specific organisms whilst inhibiting the growth of other bacterial species. For example, adding 10% sodium chloride (salt) to a general purpose medium makes it specific for the growth of *Staphylococcus* spp. If meticillin is also added this would make the medium specific for meticillin-resistant *Staphylococcus aureus* (MRSA). Using a culture medium like this improves the like-lihood and speed of isolating MRSA from clinical wound samples.

The choice of culture medium used for cultivation of bacteria from wound samples will depend on the specific preferences of the processing laboratory, and on supplied clinical details. However, they will include the following:

◆ Blood agar (incubated both aerobically and anaerobically) which is a non-selective medium and will allow the growth of all bacterial species. This gives a general picture of the total bacterial load of the specimen.

◆ MacConkey or CLED (cysteine lactose electrolyte deficient) agar. Designed to isolate faecal organisms such as *Escherichia coli*, *Pseudomonas* spp., enteric streptococci, *Proteus* spp., and so on. May indicate the level to which the wound is contaminated or colonized by the patient's own gut flora.

◆ Anaerobic selective medium designed to isolate anaerobic bacteria such as *Clostridium* spp. and *Bacteroides* spp.

◆ A variety of other selective medium, dependent upon the clinical information provided.

Bacterial growth

Bacteria are living organisms and, as such, grow and divide over time. Most bacterial species will double in number approximately every 20 minutes (this time, called the generation time, will depend on the species concerned and incubation conditions). Therefore it will take about 18 hours for the number of bacteria on a culture plate to produce visible bacterial colonies (at this point each colony will consist of several million bacterial cells). Thus bacterial culture of clinical samples takes at least 18–24 hours before results may be available. In practice, most clinical laboratories incubate their cultures for a minimum of 48 hours and sometimes for longer periods (often several days) in case there are very slow-growing organisms present in the sample.

Bacterial identification and antibiotic sensitivity testing

Following incubation, the colonies growing on the various culture media need to be identified. The colonies will vary in appearance, including size, colour, texture, and smell. Each bacterial species has a characteristic appearance on culture media and an experienced microbiologist can rapidly identify many bacterial species based on their colonial appearance.

Bacterial identification and antibiotic sensitivity tests are performed on a pure culture; therefore a single well-separated colony is selected from the culture plate; a single bacterial colony can be assumed to consist only of a single bacterial species. Most swabs from acute wounds show no bacterial growth or growth of one predominant organism. This could be the potential pathogen and is processed further to include identification and antibiotic sensitivities.

 KEY POINT

It is important to note that the recognition of possible pathogens, or other organisms of significance in the culture, depends entirely on the experience and expertise of the microbiologist. There is no automated process yet able to replace or mimic this human interpretation.

The isolate is identified using a variety of methods and assigned a scientific name; examples are *Staphylococcus aureus*, *Pseudomonas aeruginosa*, and *Escherichia coli*. Occasionally an isolate will be reported with a familiar name rather than the strict scientific one, for example, group A *Streptococcus* rather than *Streptococcus pyogenes*. Only significant bacterial isolates will appear in the final report and they will have associated antibiotic sensitivities performed. Bacterial growth that is not considered significant (e.g. skin organisms such as diphtheroid-like organisms and coagulase-negative staphylococci) is either reported as **normal skin flora** or the final report will state **No significant pathogens** isolated. Similarly, if human intestinal organisms are present then this would be reported as **mixed coliforms isolated or mixed faecal flora isolated**. Of course these organisms may also be present with recognized pathogens. This approach is taken because the body is covered with hundreds of different bacteria and most of them are part of the normal flora and non-pathogenic.

Biochemical identification of bacterial isolates

Most bacterial identification systems are based on a battery of biochemical tests using a variety of chemical substrates (see Figure 3.7). All bacteria can metabolize or degrade a large variety of chemical substances and by careful selection of the substrates it is possible to differentiate different bacterial species by virtue of the substrates utilized. These systems give a biochemical profile for each bacterial species and this profile can be compared with a database of known bacteria, thus identifying the unknown isolate. In practice, most systems use a statistical approach to identification since biochemical reactions of bacteria can vary. The identification is thus given within certain confidence limits. Bacterial identification by this process lends itself to automation and there are now several automated systems available which will identify bacteria in this way. As with culture, this method of bacterial identification requires incubation for 18–24 hours. There is therefore much interest in rapid methods of identifying important bacterial pathogens. One

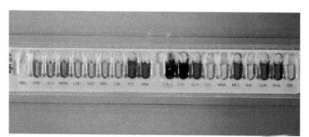

Figure 3.7 Bacterial identification: a manual commercial system based on the metabolism of chemical substrates. Each cupule contains a different substance. A suspension of the unknown organism is added to each cupule and the strip incubated overnight. The pattern of resulting positive and negative tests (indicated by a colour change) is scored numerically and this generates a seven- or eight-digit number which can be looked up in a database of known bacteria.

such rapid method is MALDI-TOF (matrix assisted laser desorption ionization time-of-flight) mass spectrometry, which will yield bacterial identifications within minutes. The equipment required for this is of considerable expense (in the region of £100,000) so this technology may only be available in large centralized laboratories. This identification technique is based on a profile of chemical markers found in the bacteria and these are unique for each species.

 KEY POINT

Occasionally, culture of a wound sample may yield no bacterial growth even after several days' incubation. There may be a number of reasons for this:

1 The patient may be on antibiotics which inhibit or kill any bacteria present in the wound.
2 The wound sample may have been collected incorrectly, or from an inappropriate part of the wound.
3 There may have been detrimental conditions during the transportation or laboratory processing of the sample, which lead to failure to isolate any organisms.
4 The wound may be sterile.

Microbiology laboratories will be fully aware of these listed conditions and will have procedures in place to mitigate as many as possible.

If a pathogen or other significant organism (sometimes more than one) is isolated from a wound sample, the processing laboratory will supply a range of antibiotic sensitivities which should guide the clinician if antibiotic therapy is thought appropriate.

Performing an antibiotic sensitivity test

The organism is suspended into sterile saline (at a concentration of approximately 10^6 colony-forming units/mL) and spread across the surface of an appropriate culture medium and a selection of antibiotics (at specific concentrations impregnated into small paper discs) are added to the surface. The plate is incubated for 18–24 hours. The diameter of the zone of inhibition is accurately measured and the results are interpreted as susceptible or resistant

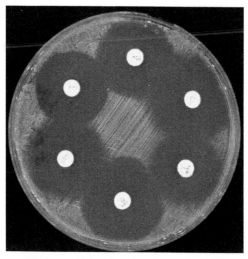

Figure 3.8 An antibiotic sensitivity plate showing zones of inhibition around discs.

Reproduced by kind permission of Don Whitley Scientific Ltd. Copyright © 2015 Don Whitley Scientific Ltd., UK.

based on the size of the zone, guided by standard methods. This is shown in Figure 3.8.

A range of antibiotic sensitivities will be reported and this will offer the clinician some choice in the selection of appropriate therapy. Factors other than organism sensitivity alone may be considered by the clinician, such as patient intolerance of an antibiotic, the cost of treatment, and so on.

The final microbiological report will collate together all the results obtained in the laboratory. These may include the following:

- The result of direct microscopic examination of the sample (Gram stain). This will indicate the groups of bacteria (if present) such as 'Gram-positive cocci', 'Gram-negative bacilli', and so on. It may also indicate the presence or absence of pus seen in the stained film.

- A list of relevant or significant organisms (which may or may not be recognized pathogens) with antibiotic sensitivities if appropriate.

- The presence of any normal or other flora present in the specimen, such as mixed faecal organisms, skin flora, and so on.

- Any comments appended to the microbiological results by the Medical Microbiologist. These may include recommended antibiotic treatment, or the need for further investigations

Traditionally, the final report described above would be a printed hard copy and this would be appended to the patient's notes. More commonly, the report will now be generated electronically.

Non-culture methods used to identify pathogens in wounds

The inevitable delay involved in the culture (isolation) of bacteria from a clinical sample is now considered to be a significant disadvantage in traditional culture methods. As a result, there is a growing demand for more rapid methods of detecting bacteria in clinical samples, and a number of these are already in common use in laboratories. Many of them rely on molecular methods such as PCR.

The polymerase chain reaction

PCR is used to amplify a specific region of DNA (usually between 0.1 and 10 kilobase pairs) which can be used to confirm detection of genes of interest from a variety of bacteria, toxins, viruses, and other organisms. The process requires several components and reagents which include the following:

+ **The DNA template** that contains the DNA target to be amplified in the patient specimen.
+ Two primers that are complementary to the DNA target.
+ An enzyme (*Taq* polymerase) that generates new DNA from all the reagents (optimum temperature 70°C).
+ **Deoxynucleoside triphosphates** (dNTPs) the building-blocks from which the DNA polymerase synthesizes a new DNA strand.
+ **Buffer solution**, providing a suitable chemical environment for optimum activity and stability of the DNA polymerase.
+ **Other buffers and essential cations**, magnesium, or manganese ions.

The PCR is commonly carried out in small volumes (10–200 µL) in small tubes in a thermal cycler, which heats and cools the tubes to achieve the temperatures required at each step of the reaction. Typically, the PCR consists of a series of 20–40 repeated temperature changes, which produces an amplified gene product.

PCR allows for rapid and highly specific diagnosis of infectious diseases, including those caused by bacteria or viruses. Many non-cultivatable or slow-growing microorganisms such as mycobacteria, anaerobes, or viruses are diagnosed by PCR rather than the traditional cultural technique.

PCR-denaturing gradient gel electrophoresis

PCR-denaturing gradient gel electrophoresis (PCR-DGGE) involves amp-lification of DNA using PCR with genus-specific primers that target 16S rDNA sequences from bacteria. Following amplification, the DNA products are separated using electrophoresis on a DGGE gel. Once separated, the seg-ments are removed from the gel, purified, and sequenced. Then the result-ant sequence is compared to a very comprehensive database and the identity given. This technique is based on the premise that the sequence of the 16s rDNA fragment is unique for each species of bacteria.

Several researchers have used molecular techniques similar to PCR-DGGE to examine the microbial ecology of chronic wounds and have iden-tified more than ten different species of bacteria in most chronic wound samples, including strict anaerobic bacteria not isolated on culture. Light and scanning electron microscopy techniques also used to analyse chronic and acute wound specimens have showed that 60% of chronic wounds con-tained a biofilm, whereas only 6% of acute wounds contained a biofilm (James et al. 2008).

There are numerous other molecular methods used in the research arena but these are not used in routine microbiology. This is because the tech-niques are either more expensive or more time-consuming compared to the traditional culture methods. Until these methods become more automated or less complex, they are unlikely to be introduced into routine diagnostic laboratories and will remain research tools.

Further reading

Ford M. *Medical Microbiology* (2nd ed). Oxford: Oxford University Press; 2014.
Standard bacteriological procedures and methods are issued by Public Health England, and give details about specimen collection and transport, laboratory methods, culture media, and so on. They are available at the following Internet site: https://www.gov.uk/government/collections/standards-for-microbiology-investigations-smi

References

Anonymous. Wound watch: three techniques for collecting wound specimens. *LPN2009*. 2008. 4(1):24–25. Available from: http://www.nursingcenter.com/lnc/static?pageid=811925

James GA, Swogger E, Wolcott R, et al. Biofilms in chronic wounds. *Wound Repair Regen*. 2008;16(1):37–44.

Levine NS, Lindberg RB, Mason AD, et al. The quantitative swab culture and smear: a quick simple method for determining the number of viable aerobic bacteria on open wounds. *J Trauma*. 1976;16(2):89–94.

Chapter 4

Acute versus chronic wounds: microbiological differences

Richard White

Objectives

On completing this chapter you should have knowledge and understanding of:

1 Acute and chronic wounds
2 The wound healing process
3 Factors impeding wound healing
4 Microorganisms associated with different wound types
5 Bacterial colonization versus infection.

Introduction to the microbiological differences between acute and chronic wounds

A wound is the result of damage to the structure of the skin and can range from a simple break in the epithelium to injury of subcutaneous tissue, with or without involvement of tendons, blood vessels, muscles, nerves, and bone. Wounds are most commonly caused by an external injury but may also be a consequence of pathological conditions, for example, vascular disease. Normal wound healing is a dynamic, complex process involving a series of co-ordinated events (Velnar et al. 2009) which can be arbitrarily divided into the four phases as outlined in Table 4.1.

Wound healing begins immediately after injury and involves an array of different cytokines and signalling molecules which are under coordinated control. Microbial interaction with any of these molecules or processes can delay wound healing and, if infection ensues, is a major cause of morbidity and mortality. A wound presents microorganisms with a potential 'ideal' environment in which to grow and divide: it is warm and moist with available nutrients. It is the combination of physical and biological characteristics of

Table 4.1 Phases of wound healing

Phase of healing	Outline of process
Phase 1 Haemostasis	Vasoconstriction and platelet aggregation
Phase 2 Inflammation	Infiltration of leucocytes, monocytes, and neutrophils. Differentiation of monocytes into macrophages
Phase 3 Proliferation	Angiogenesis
	Production of extracellular matrix
	Collagen synthesis
	Re-epithelialization
Phase 4 Remodelling	Collagen remodelling
	Maturation of the vascular system.

Source: data from Velnar T, Bailey T, and Smrkolj V. The Wound Healing Process: An Overview of the Cellular and Molecular Mechanisms. *Journal of International Medical Research*, Volume 37, Issue 5, pp.1528–42, Copyright © 2009 by SAGE Publications Ltd.

different wound types which influences the success of microbial colonization, to the detriment of the host, or the capacity of the host to withstand microbial invasion. A wound is an ecosystem, the characteristics of which will dictate microbial growth patterns, for example, exudate level (moisture), pH, tissue oxygen partial pressure, and presence of necrotic material. Added to that, the age of the wound will play a part as, over time, the resident microbial community will change. The depth of the wound is also an important factor.

Wounds are generally deemed to heal by primary intention (where the two edges are pulled and held together with sutures) or secondary intention (where the wound is allowed to heal naturally without suture). The latter, being open until healed, due to tissue loss, is the focus of this chapter.

Classification of wounds and wound types

The broad spectrum of cutaneous wounds is arbitrarily divided into two subgroups of **acute** and **chronic**, on the basis of the underlying pathophysiology and according to healing characteristics. Each subgroup has different characteristics and microbial populations, both of which can influence healing and present morbidity issues.

Acute wounds: the basics

Acute wounds are those that are newly formed (most often on healthy skin) and proceed normally through the phases of healing in a timely and orderly manner, usually ranging from 5 to 10 days, or within 30 days. They are characterized by skin that has been punctured by external means, for example, a surgical operation or traumatic wound. These wounds may also be associated with bone fractures. Acute wounds can progress to become chronic if healing does not occur within the anticipated time frame, perhaps as a result of impaired blood supply, low oxygen, reduced nutrients, or poor hygiene. Acute wounds healing by secondary intention include burns, traumatic, and some surgical excisions. It is accepted that moist wound healing is preferable for most wound types (Junker et al. 2013). The evaporative water vapour loss in grams per m² per 24 hours from intact skin is said to be ~ 200. This varies during wound healing depending upon the injury, with superficial burn levels reported at ~ 270, partial thickness burn ~ 4000, full thickness burn ~ 3500, donor site ~ 3600, and granulating (i.e. healing) wound 5000 g/m²/24 hours (Lamke 1971; Lamke and Liljedahl 1971). The levels of wound fluid (exudate) increase during the infectious process and can cause considerable problems for the patient. Exudate is similar in many respects to serum and can support a wide range of organisms including staphylococci and pseudomonads.

 DEFINITION

Exudate is the presence of wound fluid, essentially a weak aqueous solution of protein (albumin) and electrolytes, which contributes to the growth medium for microorganisms. Acute wound exudate (e.g. from a donor site) contains white blood cells, platelets, sodium, calcium and potassium cations, chloride and bicarbonate anions, glucose, and protein.

Acute wounds can be complicated by:

- Infections: whether due to contamination or poor hygiene, an infected wound will often have malodour, pus, or discoloured drainage, and is typically accompanied by pyrexia.
- Inflammation: the wound area becomes hot, red, swollen, and painful.
- Loss of function: either because of the pain or the damage caused by the wound to the affected limb or area; the loss of function can be temporary or permanent.
- Progression: in cases of delayed healing or poor wound care, acute wounds can develop to chronic wounds.

Chronic wounds

Any wound that is not healing, or one that is healing slowly, can be considered **chronic**. Chronic wounds may last for several years, and in some individuals, may never fully heal. Chronic wounds are often thought to be **stuck** in the earlier phases of wound healing (White and Cutting 2008). Typically, if a wound has not healed within 6–8 weeks, it is considered chronic and requires a different approach to wound management. There are a number of reasons why a wound will become chronic, but it is widely accepted that many of these wounds produce the correct environment for the proliferation of different microorganisms, which ultimately form a **biofilm** that enables the continuation of a stable community of bacteria that can be difficult to eradicate. Although not proven, it is likely that all chronic wounds will harbour bacteria in biofilm colonies as well as in free or 'planktonic' form (Bjarnsholt et al. 2008). Unfortunately for the patient, a chronic wound can typically produce large volumes of exudate, associated malodour and the delayed healing can always be a risk for future infection.

 KEY POINT

Causes of wound chronicity

There are many factors that contribute to the non-healing nature of chronic wounds including:

1 Advanced age of patient
2 Chronic medical conditions affecting circulation and immune functioning such as diabetes mellitus, peripheral neuropathy, peripheral arterial disease, and venous insufficiency
3 Poor nutrition
4 Impaired mobility
5 Stress
6 Poor health.

Chronic wound types

Generally, chronic wounds can be classified into one of three types:

Pressure ulcers

Once known as bedsores, these wounds are caused by prolonged, unrelieved pressure and/or shear, to an area of the body, typically over bony prominences. This constant pressure causes local ischaemia and thus inflicts damage to the skin whilst other factors, such as moisture and friction, contribute to the wound formation. These wounds typically occur in individuals who are bedridden or of limited mobility.

Arterial and venous ulcers

Venous stasis ulcers occur due to venous hypertension from dysfunctional valves in the perforator veins which causes blood to pool in the lower legs. This results in impaired venous return, extravasation of blood, and uncontrolled inflammation at the site.

Arterial insufficiency (ischaemic) ulcers are a direct result of arteriosclerosis leading to impaired perfusion of the lower leg and dorsum of the foot. If these areas are injured by trauma or pressure, the wound is unable to heal due to impaired blood flow.

Diabetic ulcers

This group includes both diabetic foot ulcers (DFUs) and ulcers of the lower limb in patients with diabetes. The important pathophysiological parameter is that of diabetes-related impairment of wound healing. This has been widely documented (Anakwenze et al. 2012; Lipsky et al. 2012; Poradzka et al. 2013) and is characterized by a reduced immune response, poor glycaemic control, elevated glycosylated haemoglobin, abnormal carbohydrate metabolism, neuropathy, deranged collagen production, and microvascular complications (Griswold 2012; Richards et al. 2012). As a result of this, opportunistic pathogens will colonize and infect DFUs (Bowling et al. 2012). In the DFU, the typical pathogen is *Staphylococcus aureus* and this can often cause osteomyelitis if left untreated.

Microbiology of acute and chronic wounds

The skin is populated with a diverse range of microorganisms and, when traumatized through an injury, is often colonized with the microorganisms found at the site of injury. Many of these organisms are non-pathogenic (incapable of causing disease) but occasionally a pathogen may gain access into the wound and may cause localized infection. The incidence of wound infection varies depending upon the site of the wound and the organism and will depend upon a number of factors including the host response and the virulence of the microorganism. Initially the microorganism has to colonize the wound (i.e. attach to the surface and reproduce) but, to cause infection, the organism has to invade local tissues. This will elicit an immune response, resulting in the well-known overt signs of infection. If the organism does not invade and does not impede healing then wound healing will occur regardless of its presence. However, it is possible that during the colonization process, additional bacterial species may enter the wound and begin to create a multispecies community, probably in the form of a biofilm, resulting in a situation where the wound will not heal, and the organisms are protected from both the host defence mechanisms, and from many antibiotics. This situation can go on ad infinitum unless the situation changes, for example, any biofilm is disrupted and healing begins, or the organisms produce such virulence factors that cause overt infection. **Biofilms** are discussed in detail in Chapter 6.

There is a marked difference in the overall microbiology of acute and chronic wounds, irrespective of the cause. Typically a single pathogen will cause an acute wound infection; however, in chronic wounds there are mixed populations of microorganisms, often existing in a biofilm (see Chapter 6). This can be confirmed *ex vivo* (but not yet *in vivo*) using scanning electron microscopy (SEM), confocal microscopy, and various diagnostic molecular techniques. Genes found in all bacteria (16S RNA) were detected, sequenced, and ultimately identified using 16S RNA databases, from samples taken from different wound types (Dowd, Sun et al. 2008) and biofilm was demonstrated using SEM. This piece of research demonstrated that 6% of acute wound infections had a biofilm, whereas 60% of chronic wounds had a biofilm. In addition, the chronic wound samples showed mixed populations of microorganisms with a number of very uncommon bacteria identified compared to conventional methods used by the majority of pathology departments. Also, this research demonstrated that the ratio of true anaerobic bacteria to facultative anaerobic bacteria altered with wound type, with pressure wounds showing higher numbers of anaerobic organisms compared to leg ulcers. Typical pathogens found in all wound types are highlighted in Box 4.1. The most common pathogen isolated from all wound

Box 4.1 Typical pathogens isolated from wounds

Gram-positive bacteria

- *Staphylococcus aureus* including MRSA
- Coagulase-negative staphylococci
- *Enterococcus* spp. including vancomycin-resistant (VRE) strains.

Anaerobic Gram-positive bacteria

- *Peptostreptococcus* spp.
- *Clostridium* spp.

Box 4.1 Typical pathogens isolated from wounds (continued)

Gram-negative bacteria

- *Pseudomonas aeruginosa*
- *Escherichia coli*
- *Klebsiella pneumoniae*
- *Serratia marcescens*
- *Enterobacter* spp.
- *Proteus* spp.
- *Acinetobacter* spp.

Anaerobic Gram-negative bacteria

- *Bacteroides* spp.
- *Prevotella* spp.

Fungi and yeasts

- *Candida* spp.
- *Aspergillus* spp.
- *Fusarium* spp.

types is *Staphylococcus aureus*. However, as previously stated, the presence of a pathogen in a wound does **not** always constitute infection. A pathogen can be present in a wound (either as a single isolate or with other organisms) without any signs of overt infection. In this case, the pathogen will be **colonizing** the wound, **not infecting** the wound.

Overt wound infection is a dynamic process and occurs when virulence factors expressed by the microorganism(s) overcome the host's immune system and produce a series of local and systemic host responses. Local responses are a purulent discharge, increased exudate, or painful spreading erythema indicative of cellulitis around a wound. Wound infection is dependent upon a number of microbial and host factors including microbial load, the blood perfusion to the wound, the general health and immune status of the host, and the virulence of the microorganism(s). The infectious process is described in detail in Chapter 2. It is important that the difference between colonization and infection is understood because it will affect the management of the wound.

> ### → DEFINITION
>
> ◆ **Colonization** occurs when microorganisms are present in a wound and are reproducing without signs of infection or impeding wound healing.
>
> ◆ **Infection** occurs when microorganisms present in a wound are actively reproducing and are producing virulence factors which overcome the host response showing overt signs of infection.
>
> ◆ **Critical colonization** occurs when microorganisms are present in the wound and are actively reproducing and have impeded wound healing without showing overt signs of infection.

Sampling the wound: quantitative versus qualitative microbiology

There is much debate on the correct sampling method for wounds with discussions on surface sampling (using the zig-zag method) compared to biopsies, and quantitative (accurate numbers) versus qualitative results (denoted as +/++ or +++, these are described in Chapter 3). The most appropriate method of sampling will be dependent upon wound type (acute or chronic), whether the wound shows signs of infection, and what information is required from the laboratory that will inform treatment. In recent years, much research has been directed at comprehensive sampling and analysis of clinical samples (Bowler and Davies, 1999; Bowler et al. 2001) by conventional microbiological methods and latterly by molecular techniques. However, a superficial wound swab will only give a representation of the superficial planktonic cells, not the biofilm. Consequently it is of limited value when sampling infected wounds (Gardner et al. 2006). The deep compartment (below the surface) of the wound must be sampled to achieve a representative picture of the microbial population (Sibbald et al. 2003). Wounds healing by secondary intent, when chronic, have a complex non-uniform bacterial ecology (Kirketerp-Moller et al. 2008) which must be considered when sampling. Technically, sampling should occur following wound bed cleansing and debridement, remembering to remove any residual antiseptics from dressings or cleansing agents prior to sampling. It is argued that tissue sampling using punch or needle aspiration biopsy approaches may be required for representative qualitative and quantitative analyses

(Bill et al. 2001; Pellizzer et al. 2001) but it must be safe to do so and not compromise the wound healing process.

In the age of molecular biology, the application of 16S ribosomal RNA gene sequencing in prokaryotes, and 18S ribosomal RNA gene sequencing in eukaryotes, has opened an entirely new vista on the diversity of the wound microbiota (Rhoads et al. 2012). Phylogenetic analysis based upon ribosomal RNA has been widely employed to define the microbiota of wounds. The range of bacteria associated with chronic wounds by 16S ribosomal RNA sequencing far exceeds that identified by 'traditional' methods (Grice and Segre 2012) see Table 4.2.

Table 4.2 Different microorganisms identified in a variety of chronic wound types using molecular techniques

Wound type	Species identified
Mixed chronic wounds	*Pseudomonas* spp., *Rhodococcus erythropolis, Actinobacterium, Staphylococcus* spp., *Pseudomonas* spp., *Haemophilus, Prevotella* spp., *Clostridium, Streptococcus, Bacteroides, Porphyromonas somerae*
Diabetic foot ulcers	*Porphyromonas, Pseudomonas, Helococcus, Varibaculum, Aerococcus, Arthrobacter, Staphylococcus, Peptoniphilus, Rhodopseudomonas, Enterococcus, Veillionella, Clostridium, Finegoldia, Haemophilus, Acinetobacter, Morganella, Serratia, Proteus, Dialister, Streptococcus, Stenotrophomonas, Peptococcus niger, Klebsiella, Actinomyces, Gordonia, Delftia, Gemella, Corynebacterium, Salmonella, Fusobacterium, Varibacterium cambriense, Enterobacter, Bacillus, Eikonella, Anaerococcus, Hydrogenophaga, Alcaligenes faecalis, Escherichia coli, Sphingomonas, Acidovorax, Prevotella, Eubacterium, Bacteroides, Selenomonadaceae, Brevibacterium, Riemerella, Bradyrhizobium, Pantoea, Abiotropica, Citrobacter, Pseudoalteromonas, Granulicatella,* and unknown bacteria
Pressure ulcers	*Peptoniphilus, Serratia, Peptococcus niger, Streptococcus, Finegoldia, Dialister, Pectobacterium, Enterobacter, Proteus, Veillionella, Clostridium, Corynebacterium striatum, Delftia, Enterococcus, Staphylococcus, Hydrogenophaga, Eggerthella, Prevotella, Varibaculum, Actinomyces europaeus, Ferrimonas, Bacillus, Fusobacterium, Alcaligenes faecalis, Riemerella, stenotrophomonas, Shewanella, Eubacterium, Anaerococcus, Dialister, Klebsiella, Porphyromonas,* and unknown bacteria

(Continued)

Table 4.2 (continued) Different microorganisms identified in a variety of chronic wound types using molecular techniques

Wound type	Species identified
Venous leg ulcers	*Enterobacter, Serratia, Stenotrophomonas, Proteus, Salmonella, Clostridium, Alcaligenes faecalis, Pseudomonas, Staphylococcus, Brevundimonas, Streptococcus, Acinetobacter, Enterococcus, Pantoea, Corynebacterium striatum, Peptoniphilus, Escherichia coli, Bacillus, Paenibacillus, Eubacterium, Klebsiella, Xanthomonas, Ferrimonas, Finegoldia, Dendrosporobacter quercicalus, Shewanella algae, Helococcus, Peptococcus, Achromobacter xylosoxidans, Shigella*, and unknown bacteria
Malignant wounds	*Staphylococcus aureus, Pseudomonas aeruginosa, Corynebacterium striatum, Proteus vulgaris. Escherichia coli, Enterococcus faecalis, Klebsiella oxytoca, Fusobaterium necrophorum, Parvimonas micra, Peptoniphilus asaccharolytica, Porphyromonas asaccharolyticus*

Source: data from Cooper RA, Bjarnsholt T, and Alhede M. Biofilms in wounds: a review of present knowledge. *Journal of Wound Care*, Volume 23, Issue 11, pp.570–82, Copyright © 2014 MA Healthcare Limited; James GA, Swogger E, Wolcott R, *et al*. Biofilms in wounds. *Wound Repair and Regeneration*, Volume 16, Issue 1, pp.37–44, Copyright © 2008 John Wiley and Sons, Inc.; Dowd SE, Sun Y, Secor PR, *et al*. Survey of bacterial diversity in chronic wounds using pyrosequencing, DGGE, and full ribosome shotgun sequencing. *BMC Microbiology*, Volume 8, pp.43, Copyright © 2008 BioMed Central Ltd.; Dowd SE, Wolcott RD, Sun Y, *et al*. Polymicriobial nature of chronic diabetic foot ulcer biofilm infections determined using bacterial tag encoded FLX amplicon pyrosequencing (bTEFAP). *PLoS One*, Volume 3, Issue 10, pp.e3326, Copyright © 2008 PLOS; Neut D, Tijdens-Creusen EJA, Bulstra SK, *et al*. Biofilms in chronic diabetic foot ulcers-a study of 2 cases. *Acta Orthopaedica*, Volume 82, Issue 3, pp.383–85. Copyright © 2011 ActaOrthop.org

Factors affecting microbial growth

Oxygen insufficiency

The degree of blood perfusion of the wound tissues (and thereby the local oxygen level) will dramatically influence growth. Therefore the organisms grown often tell us about the microclimate in the wound, and if there are high numbers of anaerobic bacteria present then the level of oxygen must be very low.

Microbiological aspects of burns

The microbiology of burns has been subject to extensive research over the past century (Church et al. 2006). This has primarily focused upon aspects of infection directly related to morbidity and mortality; consequently, complex burns have received the majority of attention. Pruitt et al. (1998) claimed that quantitative cultures are incapable of differentiating between burn wound colonization and infection, and they described histological analysis as being the most effective and rapid method for determining invasive burn wound infection.

Fungal infections in the diabetic foot

The most frequent fungal diseases are tinea pedis, onychomycosis, and candida intertrigo. Skin colonization by dermatophytes in patients with diabetes frequently leads to nail and ulcer colonization. The most frequent pathogen is *Trichophyton rubrum* (Gulcan et al. 2011).

The role of fungi in chronic wounds

It is important that fungal and yeast species are not overlooked when contemplating microbial influences on both acute and chronic wound healing. Dowd et al. (2010) have sampled over 600 patients with chronic wounds (over 900 clinical samples) obtained by sharp debridement (i.e. sampling surface and deeper tissues). Using molecular diagnostic techniques they found 208 (23%) of samples were positive for fungi. The most common species detected were *Candida* (*C. albicans*, 97/915 samples positive, 46%), followed by *Trichophyton mentagrophytes* at 32%. The authors concluded that fungi are more important pathogens than previously reported. This evidence clearly justifies more consideration than is generally afforded for fungal infection of chronic wounds.

Conclusion

Whilst much research has been directed at endogenous (neutrophil) matrix metalloproteinases (MMPs) and their role in the non-healing, chronic wound, it is important to not disregard the impact of exogenous MMPs (bacterial) on wound healing. Such enzymes are well-known virulence determinants in all tissues (Goguen et al. 1995). The common wound pathogen and biofilm-forming organism, *Pseudomonas aeruginosa*, is known to produce an elastase enzyme (invasin virulence determinant) in leg ulcers (Schmidtchen et al. 2001). This and other MMPs degrade the extracellular matrix and so interfere with the healing process through the inability for an orderly dermis to be synthesized (Wysocki et al. 2013). This enzyme and similar proteases are also produced by other wound pathogens such as *Staphylococcus aureus*, *Enterococcus faecalis*, *Proteus mirabilis*, and *Streptococcus pyogenes* and as such can degrade newly formed tissue. In addition, these enzymes can degrade antimicrobial peptides which are integral components of the innate immune system and important in prevention of colonization and infection (Schmidtchen et al. 2002).

Therefore, to conclude, microorganisms can cause devastating wound infection when invading tissues through the production of a variety of virulence factors, but equally can impede wound healing by colonizing a wound and living in a biofilm, without causing overt infection.

References

Anakwenze OA, Milby AH, Gans I, *et al.* Foot and ankle infections: diagnosis and management. *J Am Acad Orthop Surg.* 2012;**20**(11):684–693.

Bill TJ, Ratliff CR, Donovan AM, *et al.* Quantitative swab culture versus tissue biopsy: a comparison in chronic wounds. *Ostomy Wound Manage.* 2001;**47**(1):34–37.

Bjarnsholt T, Kirketerp-Møller K, Jensen PØ, *et al.* Why chronic wounds fail to heal: a novel hypothesis. *Wound Repair Regen.* 2008;**16**:1–9.

Bowler PG, Davies BJ. The microbiology of infected and noninfected leg ulcers. *Int J Dermatol.* 1999;**38**(8):573–578.

Bowler PG, Duerden BI, Armstrong DG. Wound microbiology and associated approaches to wound management. *Clin Microbiol Rev.* 2001;**14**(2):244–269.

Bowling FL, Dissanayake SU, Jude EB. Opportunistic pathogens in diabetic foot lesions. *Curr Diabetes Rev.* 2012;**8**(3):195–199.

Church D, Elsayed S, Ried O, *et al.* Burn wound infections. *Clin Micro Rev.* 2006;**19**(2):403–434.

Cooper RA, Bjarnsholt T, Alhede M. Biofilms in wounds: a review of present knowledge. *J Wound Care.* 2014;**23**(11):570–582.

Dowd SE, Hanson JD, Rees E, *et al.* Survey of fungi and yeast in polymicrobial infections in chronic wounds. *J Wound Care.* 2010;**20**(1):40–47.

Dowd SE, Sun Y, Secor PR, *et al.* Survey of bacterial diversity in chronic wounds using pyrosequencing, DGGE, and full ribosome shotgun sequencing. *BMC Microbiol.* 2008;**8**:43.

Dowd SE, Wolcott RD, Sun Y, *et al.* Polymicrobial nature of chronic diabetic foot ulcer biofilm infections determined using bacterial tag encoded FLX amplicon pyrosequencing (bTEFAP). *PLoS One.* 2008;**3**(10):e3326.

Gardner SE, Frantz RA, Saltzman CL, *et al.* Diagnostic validity of three swab techniques for identifying chronic wound infection. *Wound Repair Regen.* 2006;**14**(5):548–557.

Goguen JD, Hoe NP, Subrahmanyam YV. Proteases and bacterial virulence: a view from the trenches. *Infect Agents Dis.* 1995;**4**(1):47–54.

Grice EA, Segre JA. Interaction of microbiome and the innate immune response in chronic wounds. *Adv Exp Med Biol.* 2012;**946**:55–68.

Griswold JA. Why diabetic wounds do not heal. *Tex Heart Inst J.* 2012;**39**(6):860–861.

Gulcan A, Gulcan E, Oksuz S, *et al*. Prevalence of toenail onychomycosis in patients with type 2 diabetes mellitus and evaluation of risk factors. *J Am Podiatr Med Assoc*. 2011;**101**(1):49–54.

James GA, Swogger E, Wolcott R, *et al*. Biofilms in wounds. *Wound Repair Regen*. 2008;**16**:37–44.

Junker JP, Kamel RA, Caterson EJ, *et al*. Clinical impact upon wound healing and inflammation in moist, wet, and dry environments. *Adv Wound Care (New Rochelle)*. 2013;**2**(7):348–356.

Kirketerp-Møller K, Jensen PØ, Fazli M, *et al*. Distribution, organization, and ecology of bacteria in chronic wounds. *J Clin Microbiol*. 2008;**46**(8):2717–2722.

Lamke LO. Evaporative water loss from burns under different environmental conditions. *Scand J Plast Reconstr Surg*. 1971;**5**(2):77–81.

Lamke LO, Liljedahl SO. Evaporative water loss from burns, grafts and donor sites. *Scand J Plast Reconstr Surg*. 1971;**5**(1):17–22.

Lipsky BA, Peters EJ, Senneville E, *et al*. Expert opinion on the management of infections in the diabetic foot. *Diabetes Metab Res Rev*. 2012;**28** Suppl 1:163–178.

Neut D, Tijdens-Creusen EJA, Bulstra SK, *et al*. Biofilms in chronic diabetic foot ulcers-a study of 2 cases. *Acta Orthop*. 2011;**82**(3):383–385.

Pellizzer G, Strazzabosco M, Presi S, *et al*. Deep tissue biopsy vs. superficial swab culture monitoring in the microbiological assessment of limb-threatening diabetic foot infection. *Diabet Med*. 2001;**18**(10):822–827.

Poradzka A, Jasik M, Karnafel W, *et al*. Clinical aspects of fungal infections in diabetes. *Acta Pol Pharm*. 2013;**70**(4):587–596.

Pruitt BA Jr, McManus AT, Kim SH, *et al*. Burn wound infections: current status. *World J Surg*. 1998;**22**(2):135–145.

Rhoads DD, Cox SB, Rees EJ, *et al*. Clinical identification of bacteria in human chronic wound infections: culturing vs 16S ribosomal DNA sequencing. *BMC Infect Dis*. 2012;**12**:321–329.

Richard JL, Lavigne JP, Sotto A. Diabetes and foot infection: more than double trouble. *Diabetes Metab Res Rev*. 2012;**28** Suppl 1:46–53.

Schmidtchen A, Frick IM, Andersson E, *et al*. Proteinases of common pathogenic bacteria degrade and inactivate the antibacterial peptide LL-37. *Mol Microbiol*. 2002;**46**(1):157–168

Schmidtchen A, Wolff H, Hansson C. Differential proteinase expression by Pseudomonas aeruginosa derived from chronic leg ulcers. *Acta Derm Venereol*. 2001;**81**(6):406–409.

Serena T, Robson MC, Cooper DM, *et al*. Lack of reliability of clinical/visual assessment of chronic wound infection: the incidence of biopsy-proven infection in venous leg ulcers. *Wounds*. 2006;**18**(7):197–202.

Sibbald RG, Orsted H, Schultz GS, *et al*. Preparing the wound bed 2003: focus on infection and inflammation. *Ostomy Wound Manage*. 2003;**49**(11):24–51.

Velnar T, Bailey T, Smrkolj V. The wound healing process: an overview of the cellular and molecular mechanisms. *J Int Med Res*. 2009;**37**(5):1528–1542.

White RJ, Cutting KF. Factors involved in critical colonisation of chronic wounds. In RJ White (ed) *Advances in Wound Care* (Volume 1). Aberdeen: Wounds UK; 2008:205–219.

Wysocki AB, Bhalla-Regev SK, Tierno PM Jr, *et al.* Proteolytic activity by multiple bacterial species isolated from chronic venous leg ulcers degrades matrix substrates. *Biol Res Nurs.* 2013;**15**(4):407–415.

Chapter 5

Wound pathogens

Valerie Edwards-Jones

Objectives

On completing this chapter you should have knowledge and understanding of:

♦ The common pathogens that cause skin and soft tissue infection

♦ Their virulence mechanisms

♦ How these organisms cause skin and soft tissue infection

♦ Rare complications of infection

♦ The rarer pathogens that cause wound infection.

Introduction to wound pathogens

There are a number of bacteria that cause acute and chronic wound infections. Occasionally skin infection can also have a viral, fungal, or parasitic origin.

Normal flora of the skin

A wide variety of microorganisms exists on the skin and forms the normal flora. Higher numbers are found in the moist areas of the body, for example, the perineum, axilla, and feet. Typical bacteria found on the skin are *Micrococcus* spp., coryneforms (diphtheroids), *Staphylococcus epidermidis*, other coagulase-negative staphylococci, alpha haemolytic streptococci, and *Propionibacterium* spp. Occasionally yeasts can be found as part of the normal flora. These organisms will not usually penetrate the natural skin barrier unless it is damaged.

Common wound pathogens

Common bacterial wound pathogens can be broadly divided into Gram-positive and Gram-negative bacteria (aerobic and anaerobic) (see Table 5.1). Fungi, most commonly *Candida albicans*, may be isolated from superficial wounds and occasionally *Aspergillus* or *Mucor* spp. may be isolated from burn wounds following environmental contamination. Very occasionally viruses can cause wound infection (Bowler et al. 2001). Depending upon the pathogen, the virulence of the microorganism, and the immune response of the host, a variety of clinical symptoms may be observed. For example, *Staphylococcus aureus* frequently forms local abscesses, pus, and spreading cellulitis and *Pseudomonas aeruginosa* produces a blue/green pigment (pyocyanin) with a large amount of exudate and odour.

Table 5.1 Common bacterial wound pathogens

Gram positive	Gram negative
Aerobic/facultative anaerobic bacteria	
Staphylococcus aureus	*Escherichia coli*
Streptococcus pyogenes	*Klebsiella aerogenes*
Other streptococci (groups B, C, D, F, and G)	Other coliforms
	Pseudomonas aeruginosa
Anaerobic bacteria	
Clostridium perfringens	*Bacteroides* spp.
Peptostreptococcus spp.	

Staphylococcus aureus

Staphylococcus aureus is a facultative anaerobic, Gram-positive coccus (see Figure 5.1). It grows as a golden-coloured colony on a wide range of culture media (see Figure 5.2). It commonly colonizes the skin and can be frequently isolated from the skin, nares, axilla, and perineum as part of the normal flora. It can produce a number of different virulence factors (see Box 5.1) which account for the wide range of diseases it causes. It is the commonest pathogen isolated from both acute and chronic wounds but it is **not** always implicated in infection as not all strains of *S. aureus* possess the necessary virulence factors to cause disease.

Those strains that cause wound infection produce extracellular enzymes (hyaluronidase, collagenase, and lipase) which break down host tissues and cause invasion into deeper layers of the skin. Strains producing these enzymes will rapidly invade tissues causing local necrosis and cellulitis. *S. aureus* is well known for producing pus and also causing abscesses due to a key enzyme produced, coagulase, which breaks down fibrinogen producing a fibrin clot. This enzyme is also used in the laboratory for identification purposes as 99% of strains of *Staphylococcus aureus* produce this enzyme. When an abscess is formed, surgical drainage may be required (especially for large abscesses) as healing is unlikely unless the pus is removed.

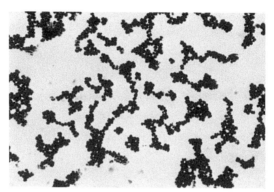

Figure 5.1 A microscopic image of *Staphylococcus aureus* stained by Gram stain. The organisms are Gram-positive so stain purple in colour. Note the individual cells form clumps not chains (compare with *Streptococcus pyogenes*).

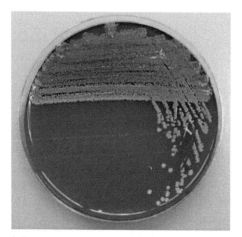

Figure 5.2 *Staphylococcus aureus* grown on Columbia blood agar. Note the smooth round colonies.

Box 5.1 *Staphylococcus aureus* virulence factors

Physical factors

- Capsule: a polysaccharide coat surrounding the bacterial cell.

Enzymes

- Coagulase: converts fibrinogen to fibrin responsible for formation of abscess.
- Hyaluronidase: breaks down hyaluronan which is a constituent of extracellular matrix.
- Collagenase: breaks the peptide bonds in collagen.
- Lipase: catalyses the hydrolysis of fats.

Toxins

- Haemolysins: alpha, beta, gamma, delta, and epsilon toxins that lyse red blood cells.
- Enterotoxins: causes vomiting and diarrhoea.
- Toxic shock syndrome toxin (TSST-1): superantigen causing overstimulation of the immune system.

S. aureus commonly causes skin infections notably, **impetigo** (infection of the epidermis) and **furunculosis** (an infection of the sweat glands). Both conditions are caused by specific strains of *S. aureus* which produce toxins locally and are characterized by a local inflammatory response and production of pus. **Impetigo** is highly infectious and spreads very easily to adjacent skin sites, distant sites on the same individual, or to the skin of other individuals. It is common in children but can also be seen in adults. A small spot quickly enlarges to a plaque-like inflamed lesion on which a yellowish exudate forms thick scabs. **Furunculosis** occurs in sebaceous glands and affects more men than women. It starts with small papules with a pointed area filled with pus which increases in size. Some papules remain blind with very red, inflamed surrounding areas. These are superficial but very painful and are treated with antibiotics, usually flucloxacillin or cephalosporins.

Complications of *Staphylococcus aureus* skin/wound infections

Certain strains of *S. aureus* can cause **scalded skin syndrome** or **Ritter's disease** in neonates, which is an extensive exfoliation of the epidermis and has the appearance of a scald. Certain strains produce exfoliatin toxins, which cause the epidermis to separate from the dermis. **Toxic shock syndrome** is a rare but life-threatening complication of *S. aureus* and unfortunately occurs in cases of **small burns** in young children. The main features are diarrhoea, rash, myalgia, hypotension, and confusion. **Always be aware of TSS** because if not treated early the fatality rate is very high because of the overactivation of the immune system by the toxin (TSST-1), and the resultant effects on multiple organs. Treatment is with antibiotics to remove the staphylococci, fluid balance, and haemodynamic support and anti-TSS antibodies from fresh frozen plasma, blood, or specific gamma globulin.

Streptococcus pyogenes (group A streptococci)

Streptococcus pyogenes (common name group A strep) is a Gram-positive facultative anaerobic coccus, growing in chains (see Figure 5.3). It commonly causes cellulitis and impetigo (along with *S. aureus)* and differentiation of streptococcal and staphylococcal cellulitis is important because the treatments differ.

If *S. pyogenes* infects an acute burn wound it will cause graft failure and has been known to produce toxins that increases the depth and severity of the burn wound. In rare cases, *S. pyogenes* can cause necrotizing fasciitis, which can be fatal if not treated promptly with radical excision and antibiotics (penicillin).

S. pyogenes produces a wide array of virulence factors including toxins and enzymes. These are described in Box 5.2. When grown on blood agar plates they produce a wide zone of beta haemolysis around the colony caused by complete lysis of the red cells (see Figure 5.4). It possesses a group A antigen on the cell surface which is used for identification purposes.

Box 5.2 *Streptococcus pyogenes* virulence factors

Physical factors

- Capsule: a hyaluronic acid-based coat surrounding the bacterial cell.
- M protein: fibrillar appendages attached to lipoteichoic acid inhibits opsonization.

Enzymes

- Streptokinase: (fibrinolysin) can dissolve fibrin clots.

Box 5.2 *Streptococcus pyogenes* **virulence factors** (continued)

- ◆ Hyaluronidase: breaks down hyaluronan which is a constituent of extracellular matrix.
- ◆ Proteinase: serine and cysteine proteinase denatures protein, serine proteinase responsible for necrotizing fasciitis.
- ◆ Nuclease: breaks down nucleic acid.

Toxins

- ◆ Haemolysins: streptolysin O and streptolysin S lyse red blood cells.
- ◆ Pyrogenic (erythrogenic toxins): four types (A, B, C, and D); cause fever, rash, and shock.
- ◆ Types A and C are superantigens and cause symptoms of streptococcal toxic shock syndrome.

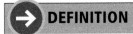 **DEFINITION**

Opsonization is a process where an antigen is prepared for phagocytosis.

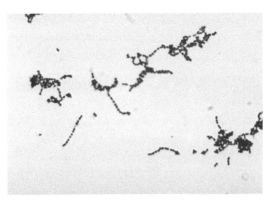

Figure 5.3 Microscopic image of *Streptococcus pyogenes* stained by Gram stain. The organisms are Gram-positive so stain purple in colour. Note the formation of chains of organisms.

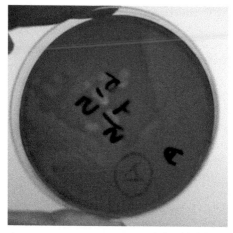

Figure 5.4 *Streptococcus pyogenes* grown on Columbia blood agar. Note the zones of haemolysis surrounding the colonies.

Reproduced by kind permission of Steve Davies. Copyright © 2015 Steve Davies.

Complications of *Streptococcus pyogenes* infections

Necrotizing fasciitis

This condition usually (but not always) follows trauma and starts with intense pain, initial cellulitis, then dusky areas appear, often with haemorrhagic bullae (blisters) (Brook and Frazier 1995). These ulcerate, revealing extensive areas of necrosis underneath which may extend along the fascia planes and abscesses may occur. Fatality is high even with treatment of penicillin and extensive surgical debridement. Necrotizing fasciitis must be distinguished from synergistic gangrene which progresses slowly and is caused by a mixture of anaerobic Gram-positive cocci and an aerobic organism.

Erysipelas

Streptococcus pyogenes can also cause **erysipelas.** Erysipelas is an intradermal infection and can be confused with cellulitis. Erysipelas nearly always affects the face or shin sites where the skin is easily traumatized. A hard, tender, erythematous lesion appears which is warm to touch and clearly demarked from the surrounding skin. If left untreated, the lesion spreads quickly and tenderness of the local lymph nodes is a common feature. Breakdown of the lymph nodes can be dangerous and lead to septicaemia. **Laboratory diagnosis** is performed by isolation of *S. pyogenes* or by serology, looking for antibodies to streptolysin O. Early diagnosis and management (using oral amoxicillin) is essential to limit the spread of infection.

Other streptococci

There are other groups of streptococci (B, C, D, and G) that may be implicated in wound infection as opportunistic pathogens. If they are isolated in pure culture from an acute wound then they should be considered as a pathogen. If found in a chronic wound as the predominant pathogen and there are associated signs of cellulitis, then again these organisms must be considered as potential pathogens. Group C and G streptococci have been implicated in necrotizing fasciitis (Bruun et al. 2013).

Pseudomonas aeruginosa

Pseudomonas aeruginosa is an opportunistic, aerobic, Gram-negative bacillus (see Figure 5.5) which is found in the human gastrointestinal tract, soil, water, and sewage. It rarely affects healthy tissue but can colonize a number of different body sites and can lead to infection, especially wounds. *P. aeruginosa* is an opportunistic pathogen and is very difficult to treat because of its natural resistance to a range of antimicrobial compounds (Wu et al. 2011). It is excellent at forming biofilms and as such can cause huge problems in healthcare environments, forming biofilms on a range of solid surfaces and pipes. It can also cause biofilms on wounds and in order to remove this from a wound, continuous cleansing, debridement, and application of appropriate antimicrobial agents are required. *P. aeruginosa* is particularly susceptible to silver compounds. *P. aeruginosa* produces a range of virulence factors (see Box 5.3) and a characteristic smell and pigment which identifies its presence in a wound (see Figure 5.6). These characteristics are also used in the laboratory as part of the identification process. It is easily isolated from a wound swab and grows readily on a wide range of culture media in the presence of oxygen.

Box 5.3 *Pseudomonas aeruginosa* virulence factors

Physical factors

- Fimbrae: used to adhere to epithelial cells.
- Slime layer (alginate): polysaccharide slime layer used to form biofilm.

Box 5.3 *Pseudomonas aeruginosa* virulence factors (continued)

Enzymes

- Elastase: cleaves collagen and elastin.
- Phospholipase and lecithinase: destroy cell membranes (all types of cell).
- Proteinase: serine and cysteine proteinase denatures protein.

Toxins

- Cytotoxin: toxic to most eukaryotic cells.
- Pyocyanin: blue/green pigment—redox active phenazine which kills by production of toxic oxygen species.

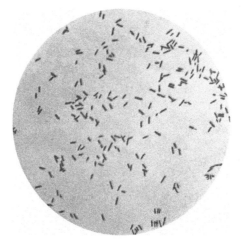

Figure 5.5 A microscopic image of *Pseudomonas aeruginosa*. Note the organisms are rod shaped and stained red by Gram stain (Gram-negative bacilli).

Reproduced from Centers for Disease Control and Prevention, Public Health Image Library (PHIL), Image ID# 2118, CDC, 1979, available from http://phil.cdc.gov/phil/details. asp?pid=2118.

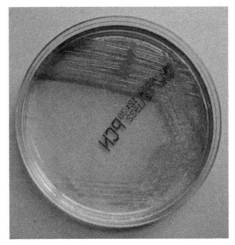

Figure 5.6 Growth of *Pseudomonas aeruginosa* on solid media showing the blue/green pigment.

Reproduced by kind permission of Steve Davies. Copyright © 2015 Steve Davies.

Coliform bacilli

This is a common term used by microbiologists for the family of bacteria known as Enterobacteriaceae. It is a group of bacteria containing over 20 different genera and over 300 different species of Gram-negative, facultative anaerobic, non-sporing bacilli. The most commonly reported organisms in this group, frequently isolated from wounds, are *Escherichia coli*, *Klebsiella* spp., *Enterobacter* spp., and *Citrobacter* spp. These organisms are found in high numbers in the human gastrointestinal tract and are frequently used by microbiologists as an indicator of faecal contamination. If found in a heavily mixed culture, these bacteria will be reported as mixed faecal flora; however, if found in pure culture or as the predominant organism in an infected wound, then the bacteria will be considered as an opportunistic pathogen and reported as such. This group of organisms does not possesses any particular virulence factors responsible for destroying tissue but in very high numbers may evoke an immune reaction in response to endotoxin that is present in their cell envelope.

In recent years, this group of bacteria have become more important because they have acquired multiple antibiotic-resistant genes (known as extended spectrum beta-lactamase producers) and are difficult to treat if the organisms get into the bloodstream.

Anaerobic organisms

Clostridium perfringens

Clostridium perfringens is an anaerobic, Gram-positive bacillus that is found in the gastrointestinal tract and environment. It is capable of producing spores that allow the organism to survive for long periods in adverse conditions. In wounds, it can cause **gas gangrene** if the environmental conditions are such that there is a lack of oxygen in the wound making it anaerobic. **Gas gangrene** is an infection of the subcutaneous tissue or muscle and is caused by a virulence factor (a powerful toxin), lecithinase, which attacks cell membranes and causes lysis of all cell types resulting in tissue destruction and killing of all macrophages, red blood cells, and platelets (immune cells). During its growth, large amounts of gas are produced which cause the typical appearance of gas gangrene. The clinical picture is that of a rapidly advancing, swollen devitalized tissue with gas and a characteristic sweet smell. Prevention is very important because it is difficult to treat without extensive debridement or amputation if it is within a limb.

Other anaerobic bacteria

Occasionally *Bacteroides* spp. (Gram-negative, anaerobic bacilli) or *Peptostreptococcus* spp. (Gram-positive, anaerobic cocci) are reported from wound cultures In pure culture, these bacteria should be considered as true pathogens but may be part of a mixed culture, which is representative of the environmental condition of the wound. These organisms cannot grow in the presence of oxygen and may be present as colonizers because of poor oxygen perfusion to the wound via the blood supply. However, if there are clinical signs of infection then these organisms must be considered as potential pathogens.

Rarer pathogens and associated infections

Erythrasma

Superficial inflammation of the creases of the skin caused by *Corynebacterium minutissimum* infection. The erythema can easily be mistaken for fungal infection or for erysipelas, but this condition is not painful and antifungal treatment is ineffective. Diagnosis is with ultraviolet light and the lesion shows characteristic salmon pink fluorescence. Treatment is with oral erythromycin or tetracycline.

Erysipeloid

Caused by the Gram-positive bacillus *Erysipelothrix rhusiopathiae*. This is a zoonotic infection from farm animals, pigs, or sheep, and is classed as an occupational hazard amongst animal workers. Initial infection presents with a dull red erythema from a puncture wound and underlying joints may become involved. Diagnosis involves a full clinical history and isolation of the Gram-positive, non-sporing bacillus. Treatment is with oral penicillins or tetracyclines.

Cutaneous mycobacterial infection

Some environmental mycobacteria can cause skin infections which fail to heal or respond to simple antibiotic treatment.

Mycobacterium marinum

Mycobacterium marinum is found in pools and rivers as well as fish aquaria. Infection occurs with colonization of traumatic skin lesions by the organism and production of indolent nodular lesions, usually on the hands. The infection can spread to the subcutaneous tissue, the fascia, and tendons. The lesions can ulcerate and produce local collections of pus. Diagnosis is by microscopy and isolation and identification of the organism (Bhatty et al. 2000). Other mycobacteria can also cause skin lesions and can occur in diabetics taking insulin. These are *Mycobacterium chelonae and Mycobacterium fortuitum.*

Buruli ulcer

Buruli ulcer is caused by *Mycobacterium ulcerans* and is characterized by a painless nodule that may turn into an ulcer which may be larger inside than at the level of the skin and may be surrounded by swelling. It commonly affects the arms or legs and occasionally bone may become involved, as the disease worsens. *M. ulcerans* releases a toxin known as mycolactone, which results in tissue death due to impairment of the immune defences. Treatment is with rifampicin and streptomycin and if treated early is successful in 80% of cases (Nakanaga et al. 2011).

Vibrio vulnificus

Vibrio vulnificus is a Gram-negative, curved, rod-shaped bacterium which is found in marine environments and coastal areas, including the Gulf of Mexico. *V. vulnificus* infection can occur though trauma from spines of fish (e.g. stingrays) or through open wounds when swimming or wading in infected waters. Infection leads to rapidly expanding cellulitis often with septicaemia and is sometimes mistaken for pemphigus. It results in disfiguring ulcers. *Vibrio vulnificus* wound infections have a mortality of approximately 25%. In patients in whom the infection produces a septicaemia, the mortality rate rises to 50%. The majority of these patients die within the first 48 hours of infection. Treatment is with third-generation cephalosporins or tetracycline (Horseman and Surani 2011).

Erythema chronicum migrans

Erythema chronicum migrans (ECM) is caused by a bite from a tick infected with a spirochaete, *Borrelia burgdorferi*. ECM is the early manifestation of Lyme disease and starts with a circular lesion which expands from the infected tick bite. Diagnosis is with immunoglobulin M antibodies to *B. burgdorferi* in the patient's serum. If left untreated, the lesion will resolve but the organism remains viable and may continue to cause problems for the patient, manifesting itself with neurological and psychological symptoms.

Further reading

Carroll KC, Brooks GF, Butel JS, *et al. Jawetz, Melnick & Adelberg's Medical Microbiology* (26th ed). New York: Lange Medical Books, McGraw Hill Education; 2013.

Goering RV, Dockrell H, Zuckerman M, *et al. Mims' Medical Microbiology* (5th ed). Philadelphia, PA: Saunders, 2013.

Murray PR, Rosenthal KS, Pfaller MA. *Medical Microbiology* (7th ed). Orlando, FL: Mosby Inc; 2013.

Todar K. *Todar's Online Textbook of Bacteriology.* Department of Bacteriology, University of Wisconsin. Available from: http://www.textbookofbacteriology.net/

References

Bhatty MA, Turner DP, Chamberlain ST. Mycobacterium marinum hand infection: case reports and review of literature. *Br J Plast Surg.* 2000;**53**:161–165.

Bowler PG, Duerden BI, Armstrong DG. Wound microbiology and associated approaches to wound management. *Clin Microbiol Rev.* 2001;**14**:244–269.

Brook I, Frazier EH. Clinical and microbiological features of necrotizing fasciitis. *J Clin Microbiol.* 1995;**33**:2382–2387.

Bruun T, Kittang BR, de Hoog BJ, *et al.* Necrotizing soft tissue infections caused by Streptococcus pyogenes and Streptococcus dysgalactiae subsp. equisimilis of groups C and G in western Norway. *Clin Microbiol Infect.* 2013;**19**(12):545–550.

Horseman MA, Surani S. A comprehensive review of Vibrio vulnificus: an important cause of severe sepsis and skin and soft-tissue infection. *Int J Infect Dis.* 2011;**15**(3):157–166.

Nakanaga K, Hoshino Y, Yotsu RR, *et al.* Nineteen cases of Buruli ulcer diagnosed in Japan from 1980 to 2010. *J Clin Microbiol.* 2011;**49**(11):3829–3836.

Wu DC, Chan WW, Metelitsa AI, *et al.* Pseudomonas skin infection: clinical features, epidemiology, and management. *Am J Clin Dermatol.* 2011;**12**:157–169.

Chapter 6

Understanding biofilms

Rose Cooper

Objectives

On completing this chapter you should have knowledge and understanding of:

1 The definition and description of a biofilm
2 Implications of immature versus mature biofilms in wound healing
3 Microorganisms living in communities
4 The role of extracellular matrix
5 Interactive effects
6 Wound biofilms
7 Treatment versus prevention of biofilms.

Introduction to biofilms

A biofilm is a new area for wound care practitioners and although well described in oral microbiology and associated with medical devices, it is still causing debate in the wound care arena. The current definition of a biofilm will be described with relevance to wounds and a number of relevant references are included should you want to read more about them.

Background

The isolation of wound pathogens has been performed routinely for more than 100 years in hospital laboratories, yet it is only recently recognized that in these artificial situations, bacteria exist in a planktonic form that is unrepresentative of their existence in natural environments where they produce copious amounts of extracellular slime (or glycocalyx) (Costerton et al. 1978). In the natural environment, bacterial cells tend to aggregate to form complex communities attached to surfaces and surround themselves with a mutually secreted polymeric matrix (Figure 6.1); these structures are known as biofilms and are widely distributed in nature and in disease (Costerton et al. 1987; Hall-Stoodley et al. 2004). Confirmation of the presence of biofilms in chronic wounds (James et al. 2008; Bjarnsholt et al. 2008; Davis et al. 2008) has altered perceptions on managing these wounds.

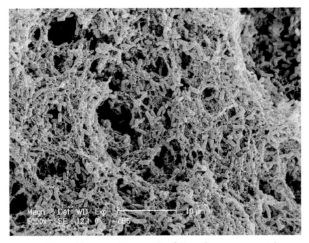

Figure 6.1 Scanning electron micrograph of *Pseudomonas aeruginosa* cultivated on a coverslip.

 KEY POINT

A **wound biofilm** is a coherent community of aggregated microorganisms encased within an extracellular matrix of polymeric substances (EPS) that is associated with a cutaneous wound.

Evidence of biofilms in wounds

The first evidence of biofilms in wounds came from sutures and staples removed from ten healed surgical wounds where several types of bacteria embedded in fibrous, extracellular material were observed using electron microscopy although only *Staphylococcus epidermidis* was isolated in every case (Gristina et al. 1985). All of the wounds had healed without evidence of infection and inflammation, indicating that biofilms do not always have adverse effects. Biofilms have since been associated with in-dwelling medical devices and have been implicated in recurrent infections (Donlan 2001).

FACT

During the past 40 years, a link has emerged between biofilms and persistent diseases such as cystic fibrosis, endocarditis, kidney stones, prostatitis, periodontal disease, dental caries, and otitis media (Potera 1999; Parsek and Singh 2003).

Historically, experiments with animal models showed that biofilms could form in acute wounds (Akiyama et al. 1993, 1994, 2002; Serralta et al. 2001), and wound pathogens (such as *Staphylococcus aureus* and *Pseudomonas aeruginosa*) have been grown as biofilms in the laboratory (Akiyama et al. 1994; Harrison-Balestra et al. 2003).

Three landmark studies proved unequivocally that biofilms develop in wounds (Bjarnsholt et al. 2008; Davis et al. 2008; James et al. 2008). Using scanning electron microscopy (SEM) of biopsies collected from 50 chronic wounds, the presence of large aggregates of bacteria predominantly containing Gram-positive cocci embedded in amorphous extracellular material (EPS) was found in 60% of specimens. Biofilms of Gram-negative bacteria, as well as mixed-species biofilms, were observed in specimens from chronic wounds; however, only one of the 16 acute wound specimens had a biofilm. Thus wound chronicity and the presence of biofilm was shown to be associated (P <0.001) (James et al. 2008). Additionally molecular analysis of selected chronic wound samples demonstrated the presence of diverse polymicrobial communities that contained anaerobic species that were not detected by conventional culturing methods (James et al. 2008).

In another study, fluorescence *in situ* hybridization (FISH) with peptide nucleic acid (PNA) probes was used to identify and locate specific bacteria directly in sections of chronic wound specimens. Single cells of *P. aeruginosa* were observed in one section, and microcolonies (or biofilms) of either cocci or *P. aeruginosa* in other sections. Importantly bacterial aggregates surrounded but not penetrated by host cells were observed (Bjarnsholt et al. 2008).

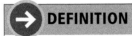

DEFINITION

- **Scanning electron microscopy (SEM)** is a type of electron microscopy where images are produced by scanning the surface with a focused beam of electrons.

- **Molecular analyses** are techniques for looking for genes or pieces of DNA, for example, PCR or DGGE; these are described further in Chapter 3.

- **Fluorescence *in situ* hybridization (FISH)** is a technique where fluorescent probes are used to detect DNA in thin sections of tissue removed from a patient. These probes can be visualized using fluorescent microscopy.

- **Microcolonies** are colonies of bacteria that can only be observed using a microscope.

Insight into the role for biofilms in wound colonization and infection came from research carried out using a porcine model with partial-thickness wounds inoculated with a culture of *Staphylococcus aureus*. Fifteen wounds were treated with one of two topical antibiotic preparations either 15 minutes after inoculation (to mimic a planktonic infection) or 48 hours after inoculation (to allow a biofilm to establish). Light microscopy, SEM, and epifluorescence microscopy (EpiFM) were used to monitor effects. Untreated wounds showed aggregated microcolonies of staphylococci attached to the wound bed and embedded in amorphous extracellular material (a biofilm), but wounds treated shortly after inoculation with *S. aureus* had no biofilm, showing that both antibiotic treatments eliminated planktonic bacteria and prevented biofilm formation. Wounds where biofilms were allowed to establish before antibiotic treatment were not eradicated, showing that bacteria in established wound biofilms were less susceptible to antibiotics than planktonic bacteria (Davis et al. 2008).

The distribution of biofilms in chronic wounds is uneven which makes wound sampling problematic. In a study in 2008, biopsies taken from chronic wounds suspected of being colonized by *P. aeruginosa* were examined by conventional culturing technique and by FISH. *S. aureus* was isolated more often than *P. aeruginosa*, even though biofilms with *P. aeruginosa* embedded in alginate (an extracellular polysaccharide substance secreted by *P. aeruginosa*) were visualized by FISH in 70% of wounds (showing no correlation of techniques). Another study showed *S. aureus* was located closer to the wound bed surface than *P. aeruginosa* (Kirketerp-Møller et al. 2008) and this differential organization of multispecies biofilms within a wound was confirmed in chronic wounds where *P. aeruginosa* aggregates were located at distances significantly distant from the wound bed surface than *S. aureus* biofilms (Fazli et al. 2009).

Biofilms have also been identified in an uninfected chronic leg ulcer (Malic et al. 2009), burns (Kennedy et al. 2010), and in diabetic foot ulcers (Neut et al. 2011) using FISH and EpiFM.

Biofilm development

Many systems have been developed for investigating the events of biofilm formation in the laboratory and in animals. To date, the formation of *P. aeruginosa* biofilms has been studied most frequently *in vitro* and are represented in a diagrammatic illustration (Figure 6.2).

> 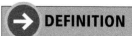 **DEFINITION**
>
> *In vitro* refers to the study of organisms within the laboratory, outside of their normal biological environment.

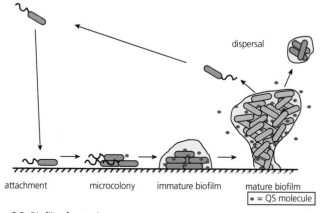

Figure 6.2 Biofilm formation.

> **KEY POINT**
>
> The process of biofilm formation can be divided into three stages: **attachment**, **maturation**, and **dispersal** (Sauer et al. 2002; Klausen et al. 2003).

Attachment

Single-celled planktonic bacteria use their flagella to swim towards a solid surface where nutrients tend to be more concentrated. **Motility** over the moist surface is switched to **twitching**, which is achieved using type IV pili. Initially bacteria adhere reversibly to the surface, but eventually the cells become irreversibly attached to the surface. The cells are described as being sessile at this stage. They reproduce to form a microcolony and start to secrete extracellular polymers.

 DEFINITION

- ◆ A **flagellum** is an appendage (consisting of protein) on the bacterial cell surface that is used for propulsion.

- ◆ A **pilus** is an appendage on the bacterial cell surface that is used for adhesion.

Maturation

From this point, biofilm development is tightly regulated by complex changes in gene expression that are controlled by cell–cell communication (otherwise known as quorum sensing (QS)) which ensures a coordinated population response (O'Toole et al. 2000; Stoodley et al. 2002). Environmental factors also influence the maturation of a biofilm.

 KEY POINT

Quorum sensing (QS) is the production and detection of signalling molecules, also known as autoinducers; these highly specific cell–cell signalling molecules are peptide molecules in Gram-positive bacteria and lactones in Gram-negative bacteria. The transition from planktonic cells within a microcolony to cells within a mature biofilm depends on continued growth and division of bacterial cells until a critical cell density (or quorum) is reached. This is recognized in each species by the detection of a threshold density of their own autoinducer molecules. Thus size of the population density for each microbial species within the biofilm community is reflected in the quantity of QS molecules produced and detected.

Differential expression of genes within biofilm subpopulations leads to the formation of irregular three-dimensional stacks interspersed by fluid-filled accessory channels as cells move away from the attachment site by twitching. One important outcome of QS during biofilm maturation is the upregulation and production of virulence determinants when the quorum is reached (Nakagami et al. 2011). Cells in mature biofilms exhibit virulence markers not detected in cells located within an immature biofilm. In *P. aeruginosa*, for example, production of rhamnolipid, elastase, exotoxins A and S, alkaline protease, phospholipases, siderophores, pyocyanin, and some surface proteins that bind sugars are switched on when high density populations are reached. This is also seen in mature biofilms of *S. aureus* where many surface adhesins and exotoxins are detected.

Soluble products produced by *S. aureus* in culture have been shown to elicit different responses in keratinocytes, with biofilm cells inducing a marked inflammatory response compared to planktonic cells (Secor et al. 2011).

One significant change seen in some cells within the mature biofilm is that growth rates are diminished and this impacts on their antimicrobial susceptibility. Many antimicrobial agents target biosynthetic pathways, and are most effective in rapidly growing cells. Increased resistance of bacteria in biofilms compared to planktonic bacteria has been reviewed for antibiotics (Stewart and Costerton 2001) and for disinfectants (Bridier et al. 2013).

Dispersal

Dispersal of cells from a mature biofilm is not entirely understood, although it has been suggested to be a programmed event (Stoodly et al. 2001). It is possible that single cells can swim away to colonize other sites, mass migration can occur, or biofilm fragments can become detached by shear forces.

Biofilms comprised of mixed species are common in nature and co-aggregation of different microbial species is thought to be important in the development of a multispecies biofilm (Rickard et al. 2003). The first cells to attach to a surface are known as primary colonizers (or pioneers) and interactions between protein molecules on the surface of one type of microbe (adhesins) and sugars (receptors) on the surface of another allows secondary colonizers to join the growing aggregate. Further co-aggregation leads to species diversity within the biofilm (Figure 6.3). The differential spatial organization of *S. aureus* and *P. aeruginosa* observed in some chronic wounds indicates that single-species biofilms can also exist in chronic wounds.

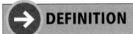

DEFINITION

Co-aggregation is the process of cell-to-cell recognition and attachment using specific molecules.

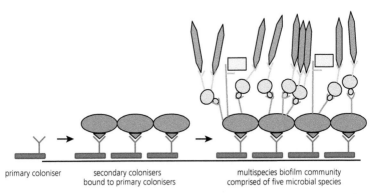

primary coloniser   secondary colonisers   multispecies biofilm community
                     bound to primary colonisers   comprised of five microbial species

Figure 6.3 The role of co-aggregation in the formation of a biofilm.

KEY POINT

Biofilms can exist as a single-species biofilm (e.g. *P. aeruginosa* biofilm) and also as multispecies biofilms (e.g. *P. aeruginosa, S. aureus,* and other bacteria biofilm)

Many bacteria isolated from wounds can form a single-species biofilm in laboratory conditions and tissue-engineered skin has been used to study biofilm development *in vitro* (Charles et al. 2009). How accurately these models reflect biofilm formation and behaviour in wounds *in vivo* is not yet known, nor how many aggregated cells in a wound represent a mature biofilm.

The role of extracellular matrix

All mature biofilms are surrounded by a complex, slimy extracellular matrix, which is vital for survival. The EPS scaffold defines biofilm architecture and varying chemical and physical gradients within the differing regions of biofilm EPS allow a range of microhabitats to become populated by physiologically diverse cells (Sutherland 2001). Another advantage is that cells held in close proximity to one another may cooperate metabolically in the collective degradation of unusual substrates and are readily able to exchange genetic material. Because EPS is produced by biofilm cells, its composition varies with species and location. It is largely made up of water (up to 97%) and polysaccharides, with proteins, lipids, extracellular DNA (eDNA), and RNA present in smaller proportions.

Numerous polysaccharides from EPS have been characterized (Bales et al. 2013); constituent sugars include mannose, galactose, glucose, N-acetylglucosamine, galacturonic acid, and polymers including glucans, fructans, cellulose, xanthan, and alginate. Alginate contributes to biofilm structure, helps to prevent ingress of phagocytes, binds cationic inhibitors such as aminoglycosides, and mops up free radicals.

Proteins in EPS include extracellular enzymes which function in extracellular digestion of complex molecules, thus providing a ready supply of nutrients for the biofilm. Some of these enzymes help in biofilm survival by digesting EPS in times of starvation. Proteins may also contribute to biofilm structure.

It has been shown that eDNA released from lysed cells, contributes to biofilm adhesion, stability, structural strength, and protection against antimicrobial agents (Whitchurch et al. 2002). It also facilitates efficient movement of twitching cells within a biofilm (Gloag et al. 2013).

 KEY POINT

EPS is crucial to biofilm structure and function and it confers many benefits to constituent biofilm members (Flemming and Wingender 2010). These benefits include the following:

◆ Adhesion
◆ Structural organization of aggregated cells
◆ Water retention
◆ Acts as a protective barrier
◆ Uptake of materials from the environment
◆ Source of nutrients
◆ Reservoir of enzymes, genetic material, and exported products.

Immune evasion by microbial cells within mature biofilms

Chronic wounds are characterized by elevated levels of pro-inflammatory cy-tokines, proteases, free radicals, unresponsive/senescent cells, and decreased levels of growth factors (Mast et al. 1996). Massive infiltration of pressure ulcers by polymorphonuclear neutrophils (PMN) was observed by light mi-croscopy and linked to wound chronicity (Diegelmann 2003). Using FISH and EpiFM, microcolonies of *P. aeruginosa* in chronic wound biopsies were found to be surrounded, but not permeated by PMNs. In laboratory experi-ments, FISH and confocal laser scanning microscopy (CLSM) were used to demonstrate that PMNs penetrated microcolonies of *P. aeruginosa* mutants that were deficient in QS molecules but remained outside microcolonies of *P. aeruginosa* with fully functional QS (Bjarnsholt et al. 2008). *P. aeruginosa in vitro* was shown to be protected from the phagocytic effects of PMNs by the production of rhamnolipid under the control of QS which caused rapid lysis of PMNs (Jensen et al. 2007). The production of rhamnolipid was pos-tulated to be the mechanism utilized by *P. aeruginosa* to avoid clearance in chronic wounds (Bjarnsholt et al. 2008). Supportive evidence for the role of *P. aeruginosa* in cellular inflammation came from enumerating neutrophils in biopsy specimens from chronic venous leg ulcers with FISH and CLSM (Fazli et al. 2011) and from a chronic wound model in a mouse (Trøstrup et al. 2013). The presence of *P. aeruginosa* in chronic wounds, therefore, is considered to be an important factor in the development of a chronic inflam-matory response and impaired healing.

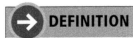 **DEFINITION**

Confocal laser scanning microscopy (CLSM) is a technique where lasers are used to produce a high-resolution optical image with depth selectivity.

Inability of leucocytes to infiltrate mature *S. aureus* biofilms *in vitro* has also been reported (Leid et al. 2002) and impaired healing due to *S. aureus* bio-films by delaying re-epithelialization in a murine model has been observed (Schierle et al. 2009). The precise mechanisms for these effects are not yet known.

It has been suggested that biofilms continually release small numbers of planktonic bacteria to perpetuate the inflammatory response and that subsequent lysis of neutrophils provides a source of nutrients for cells within the biofilm.

Diagnosing wound biofilms

Methods to detect biofilms in wound tissue have not yet been validated but a number of research methods are currently in use.

In certain natural environments, where biofilms have established in undisturbed locations for a considerable time, it may be possible to detect slimy structures (e.g. within water pipes) but microscopic confirmation is required to confirm a suspicion of biofilms and wounds are no exception. Sloughy wounds may appear slimy, but this does not necessarily indicate the presence of a biofilm. Slough has been defined as 'A mixture of dead white cells, dead bacteria, rehydrated necrotic tissue and fibrous tissue' (Collins et al. 2002).

When wound swabs or biopsies are processed in routine medical microbiology laboratories, recovered species grow planktonically as isolated colonies, not as biofilms. Therefore it is not possible to deduce whether a biofilm might have been present in that wound by observing the morphology of recovered cultures. The choice of specimen collected from a wound also influences laboratory observations. The adherence of biofilms to surfaces limits their removal by swabbing, and biofilms located in deep tissue will only be removed in biopsies. Until standardized methods of recovering and detecting biofilms are developed, routine testing is not possible. At present it is only in specialized, research laboratories that attempts to identify biofilms in wounds have been made.

KEY POINT

Techniques used to detect biofilms in wounds to date include:

◆ Scanning electron microscopy (SEM)

◆ Epifluorescent microscopy (EpiFM)

◆ Confocal laser scanning microscopy (CLSM)

◆ Detection of quorum sensing molecules (QS)

◆ Molecular characterization of species present.

Of the studies published to date to confirm the presence of biofilms in specimens collected from chronic wounds, three utilized SEM (James et al. 2008; Davis et al. 2008; Kennedy et al. 2010). This technique allowed communities of mixed species to be observed relatively easily without identifying specific organisms.

EpiFM has been used to characterize biofilms in chronic wounds by staining EPS with calcofluor white (Davis et al. 2008; Neut et al. 2011) and by identifying specific bacteria by staining with peptide nucleic acid (PNA) probes (Bjarnsholt et al. 2008). The advantage of using CLSM with fluorescent staining is that sections within the specimen at differing depths can by visualized and the images re-constructed to show the three-dimensional structure of the biofilm (Kirketerp-Møller et al. 2008; Malic et al. 2009; Fazli et al. 2009; Neut et al. 2011). This approach is limited to the availability of specific PNA probes that emit fluorescence of differing light for each microbial species sought (Figure 6.4).

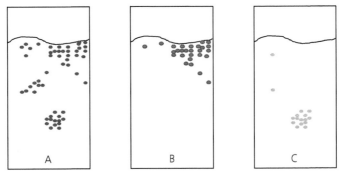

Figure 6.4 Differential staining of a biopsy. (A) Biopsy stained with a universal fluorescent bacterial probe; (B) biopsy stained with S. aureus probe; (C) biopsy stained with *Pseudomonas aeruginosa* probe.

Detection of autoinducers (QS molecules) is an indirect method of detecting biofilms but this is a research tool and not suitable for routine diagnostic laboratories. QS molecules of *P. aeruginosa* were detected in infected ischaemic wound in rats but not in uninfected wounds (Nakagami et al. 2008), and in 15 of 30 chronic wound samples detectable levels of QS were found (Rickard et al. 2010).

The molecular characterization of species in chronic wounds began with a diabetic foot ulcer (Redkar et al. 2000) and it soon became evident that slow growing or fastidious organisms that were difficult to cultivate and identify by routine methods were being underestimated in wound specimens (Davies et al. 2001; Hill et al. 2003; Dowd et al. 2008). In one study, several molecular approaches were used to investigate the diversity of bacterial flora in the biofilms within samples derived from three types of chronic wounds (Dowd, Sun et al. 2008). *Staphylococcus, Pseudomonas, Peptoniphus, Enterobacter, Stenotrophomonas, Finegoldia*, and *Serratia* were found to be common to all wounds, with facultative Gram-negative rods most frequently detected in venous leg ulcers and to a lesser extent in diabetic foot ulcers, and strict Gram-positive cocci anaerobes most frequently detected in pressure ulcers. Compared to molecular techniques, conventional culture correctly identified the main bacteria in only one of 30 patients tested (Dowd, Sun et al. 2008).

The polymicrobial flora of biofilms in each of the following wounds has now been characterized: chronic diabetic foot ulcers, chronic venous leg ulcers, surgical site infections, and malignant wounds (Dowd, Wolcott et al. 2008; Oates et al. 2012; Thomsen et al. 2010; Wolcott et al. 2009; Fromantin et al. 2013, respectively). Yeasts and fungi have also been diagnosed in chronic wounds using these new technologies (Leake et al. 2009; Dowd, Delton Hanson et al. 2011). An indication of the relative sensitivity of identification procedures was illustrated when conventional culturing of 168 wound specimens identified 17 different bacteria versus 338 different taxa identified with molecular methods (Rhoads et al. 2012). At present, molecular characterization of wound samples requires specialist facilities and dedicated staff, but can yield results in shorter intervals than cultures in an optimized set-up. It does not, however, necessarily provide comprehensive antibiotic sensitivity data, demonstrate bacterial viability, or distinguish between planktonic and biofilm cells.

Treatment and prevention of biofilms in wounds

Wound infections due to planktonic bacteria usually respond to appropriate antibiotic therapy. Biofilms are especially difficult to treat, sometimes up to 1000 times less susceptible than the planktonic equivalents (Stewart and Costerton 2001; Bridier et al. 2013). Permanent genetic mutations that confer antibiotic and antiseptic resistance are often absent from cells in biofilms and the ability to withstand antimicrobial agents is likely to be due to physiological adaptations. This is described as antimicrobial tolerance, and although the mechanisms are not completely understood, it has been attributed to many factors including reduced penetration of antimicrobial agents through the EPS matrix due to sequestration of positively charged molecules, deactivation of antimicrobials within surface layers, limited diffusion of negatively charged antibiotics, and reduced microbial growth rates due to oxygen or nutrient limitations. A small proportion of the bacterial cells within the biofilm (< 1%) are known as 'persister cells' which explain recurrent infections that often characterize biofilm infections (Spoering and Lewis 2001). Persister cells are shielded from immune responses and the effects of antimicrobials by being located deep within a biofilm. The concept of persisters was postulated by Bigger (1944) who noted that in soldiers injured during World War II, wound infections treated with penicillin sometimes showed temporary resolution of infection with a recurring infection later.

Strategies to control wound biofilms can be divided into three categories according to the stage in the biofilm development cycle: prevention of attachment, interference with QS, or disruption of the established biofilm. Mature biofilms will probably require a combined antimicrobial assault, rather than a single intervention.

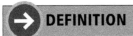

DEFINITION

- **Sequestration** is the biological process through which an organism accumulates a compound.
- **Persister cells** are slow-growing or dormant cells that seem to increase in stressed conditions (e.g. nutrient-limited environments or in the presence of antimicrobial agents) and decrease in conditions that favour rapid growth.

Prevention of attachment

Lactoferrin prevents biofilm formation by sequestering iron, which impacts on bacterial motility, and by disrupting the permeability of the outer membrane of Gram-negative bacteria (Weinberg 2004). Xylitol binds to the surface of Gram-positive bacteria to block adherence to host tissue (Tapiainen et al. 2004). Manuka honey interferes with adherence of *Streptococcus* (Maddocks et al. 2012) and *P. aeruginosa* (Roberts et al. 2012).

Interference with quorum sensing

Preventing cell–cell communication by interfering with QS seems to offer real potential in controlling biofilms. One candidate molecule suggested so far is honey (Wang et al. 2012).

Disruption of an established biofilm

Removal of biofilm by sharp debridement is an effective way of disrupting the biofilm and reducing bacterial numbers in wounds and to prepare the wound bed, but it will not remove all biofilm cells and residual cells will allow the biofilm to reform later. Therefore following debridement, application of topical antimicrobials that further reduce organism numbers or enzymes that degrade components of the EPS are required. Variidase (otherwise known as streptodornase) has been shown to disrupt *P. aeruginosa* biofilms *in vitro* by targeting eDNA (Nemoto et al. 2003) and maggot secretions contain proteolytic enzymes which are able to degrade components in EPS to destabilize biofilm integrity (Chambers et al. 2003). Generation of hydrogen peroxide by glucose oxidase and lactoperoxidase has been shown to disrupt biofilms *in vitro* (Johansen et al. 1997; Cooper 2013). Manuka honey also disrupts biofilms *in vitro* (Maddocks et al. 2012; Roberts et al. 2012; Cooper et al. 2014).

The ability of silver to disrupt established biofilms has been tested in laboratory models, with some conflicting results (Chaw et al. 2005; Bjarnsholt et al. 2007; Percival et al. 2007, 2008). Testing of a range of antimicrobial dressings in a sophisticated laboratory model showed complete and efficient killing of biofilms by each of cadexomer iodine and povidone iodine, in contrast to the other dressings (Hill et al. 2010).

However, there is little clinical evidence yet to demonstrate efficacy of any of these antibiofilm strategies. One novel approach was developed following the demonstration in four laboratory models that biofilms were more susceptible to antimicrobial agents during the first 24 hours of formation than mature biofilms (Wolcott et al. 2010). Hence removal of a mature biofilm by sharp debridement followed by topical antibiotics targeted at those microbial species previously identified within that wound by molecular analysis has been suggested to be a valid means to prevent the reformation of the biofilm by inhibiting the biofilm community at its most susceptible stage when trying to re-establish. This has been called biofilm-based wound care (BBWC) and was first employed in a clinical study where 190 patients with critical limb ischaemia were managed by sharp debridement (plus ultrasonic debridement in some cases) followed by topical treatment with lactoferrin and xylitol, and silver-impregnated dressings, or cadexomer iodine, or antibiotics (Wolcott and Rhoads 2008). Compared to a previous study, improved healing outcomes were recorded, even for patients with osteomyelitis (Wolcott and Rhoads 2008). Similarly biofilm suppression by BBWC was shown to improve the wound bed to increase the efficacy of cell-based therapy with grafts (Wolcott and Cox 2013). The benefits of a personalized cocktail of antibiotics selected following molecular diagnosis of patients' wounds have been demonstrated in a retrospective study (Dowd, Wolcott et al. 2011).

Future antibiofilm therapies may include electrical stimulation, QS inhibitors, and bacteriophage.

KEY POINT

The characteristics of cells within a mature biofilm include the following:

- Adherent cells embedded within a complex EPS
- Physiological and metabolic functions distinct from planktonic cells
- Diversity of physiological and metabolic functions within subpopulations of cells
- Increased virulence
- Increased capacity to evade host immune responses
- Increased tolerance to antimicrobial agents.

These attributes contribute to the persistence of biofilms in wounds, and help to explain difficulties in their diagnosis and their undesirable impact on the patient.

KEY POINT

There are numerous advantages for microbial species to exist within a biofilm (Jeffersen 2004):

- Stable colonization of a nutrient-rich environment
- Protection from host immune responses
- Tolerance to antimicrobial agents
- Access to the cooperative benefits of the biofilm community.

Conclusion

It is clear that innovative management strategies must be developed and that an understanding of the behaviour of biofilms is an essential prerequisite for further advances. Developing better treatment options will depend not only on finding novel biofilm inhibitors, but in gathering clinical evidence on their efficacy with the aid of rapid, routine biofilm detection methods. Standardized methods to evaluate antibiofilm treatments are needed and there is much research to complete before biofilms in wounds will truly be conquered. However, before biofilms were discovered in wounds, it should be noted that chronic wounds were not always managed without success.

References

Akiyama H, Huh WK, Yamasaki O, et al. Confocal laser scanning microscopic observation of glycocalyx by Staphylococcus aureus in mouse skin: does S. aureus generally produce a biofilm on damaged skin? Br J Dermatol. 2002;147(5):879–885.

Akiyama H, Kanzaki H, Abe Y, et al. Staphylococcus aureus infection on experimental croton oil-inflamed skin. J Dermatol Sci. 1994;8(1):1–10.

Akiyama H, Torigoe R, Arata J. Interaction of Staphylococcus aureus cells and silk thread in vitro and in mouse skin. J Dermatol Sci. 1993;6(3):247–257.

Bales PM, Renke EM, May SL, et al. Purification and characterization of biofilm-associated EPS exopolysaccharides from ESKAPE organisms and other pathogens. PLoS One. 2013;8(6):e67950.

Bigger JW. Treatment of staphylococcal infections with penicillin by intermittent sterilization. Lancet. 1944;ii:497–500.

Bjarnsholt T, Kirketerp-Møller K, Jensen PØ, et al. Why chronic wounds will not heal: a novel hypothesis. Wound Repair Regen. 2008;16(1):2–10.

Bjarnsholt T, Kirketerp-Møller K, Kristiansen S, et al. Silver against Pseudomonas aeruginosa biofilms. APMIS. 2007;115(8):921–928.

Bridier A, Briandet R, Thomas V, et al. Resistance of bacterial biofilms to disinfectants: a review. Biofouling. 2013;27(9):1017–1032.

Chambers L, Woodrow S, Brown AP, et al. Degradation of extracellular matrix components by defined proteinases from the greenbottle larvae Lucilia sericata used for the clinical debridement of non-healing wounds. Br J Dermatol. 2003;148(1):14–23.

Charles CA, Ricotti CA, Davis SC, et al. Use of tissue engineered skin to study in vitro biofilm development. Dermatol Surg. 2009;35(9):1334–1341.

Chaw KC, Manimaran M, Tay FEH. Role of silver ions in destabilization of intermolecular adhesion forces measured by atomic force microscopy in Staphylococcus epidermidis biofilms. Antimicrob Agents Chemother. 2005;49(12):4853–4859.

Collins F, Hampton S, White R. A–Z Dictionary of Wound Care. Wiltshire: Mark Allen Publishing Ltd; 2002.

Cooper RA. Inhibition of biofilms by glucose oxidase, lactoperoxidase and guaiacol: the active antibacterial component in an enzyme alginogel. Int Wound J. 2013;10(6):630–637.

Cooper RA, Jenkins L, Hooper S. Inhibition of Pseudomonas aeruginosa biofilms by Medihoney™. *J Wound Care.* 2014;**23**(3):93–104.

Costerton JW, Cheng K-J, Geesey GG, *et al.* Bacterial biofilms in nature and disease. *Annu Rev Microbiol.* 1987;**41**:435–464.

Costerton JW, Geesey GG, Cheng KJ. How bacteria stick. *Sci Am.* 1978;**238**(1): 86–95.

Davies CE, Wilson MJ, Hill KE, *et al.* Use of molecular techniques to study microbial diversity in the skin: chronic wounds reevaluated. *Wound Repair Regen.* 2001;**9**(5):332–340.

Davis SC, Ricotti C, Cazzaniga A, *et al.* Microscopic and physiologic evidence for biofilm-associated wound colonization in vivo. *Wound Repair Regen.* 2008;**16**(1):23–29.

Diegelmann RF. Excessive neutrophils characterize chronic pressure ulcers. *Wound Repair Regen.* 2003;**11**(6):490–495.

Donlan RM. Biofilms and device-associated infections. *Emerg Infect Dis.* 2001;**7**(2): 277–281.

Dowd SE, Delton Hanson J, Rees E, *et al.* Survey of fungi and yeast in polymicrobial infections in chronic wounds. *J Wound Care.* 2011;**20**(1):40–47.

Dowd SE, Sun Y, Secor PR, *et al.* Survey of bacterial diversity in chronic wounds using pyrosequencing, DGGE, and full ribosome shotgun sequencing. *BMC Microbiol.* 2008;**8**:43.

Dowd SE, Wolcott RD, Kennedy J, *et al.* Molecular diagnostics and personalised medicine in wound care: assessment of outcomes. *J Wound Care.* 2011;**20**(5):232, 234–239.

Dowd SE, Wolcott RD, Sun Y, *et al.* Polymicrobial nature of chronic diabetic foot ulcer biofilm infections determined using bacterial tag encoded FLX amplicon pyrosequencing (bTEFAP). *PLoS One.* 2008;**3**(10):e3326

Fazli M, Bjarnsholt T, Kirketerp-Møller K, *et al.* Non-random distribution of Pseudomonas aeruginosa and Staphylococcus aureus in chronic wounds. *J Clin Microbiol.* 2009;**47**(12):4084–4089.

Fazli M, Bjarnsholt T, Kirketerp-Møller K, *et al.* Quantitative analysis of the cellular inflammatory response against biofilm bacteria in chronic wounds. *Wound Repair Regen.* 2011;**19**(3):387–391.

Flemming H-C, Wingender J. The biofilm matrix. *Nat Rev Microbiol.* 2010;**8**(9):623–633.

Fromantin I, Seyer D, Watson S, *et al.* Bacterial floras and biofilms of malignant wounds associated with breast cancers. *J Clin Microbiol.* 2013;**51**(10): 3368–3373.

Gloag ES, Turnbull L, Huang A, *et al.* Self-organization of bacterial biofilm is facilitated by extracellular DNA. *Proc Natl Acad Sci U S A.* 2013;**110**(28):11541–11546.

Gristina AG, Price JL, Hobgood CD, *et al.* Bacterial colonisation of percutaneous sutures. *Surgery.* 1985;**98**(1):12–19.

Hall-Stoodley L, Costerton JW, Stoodley P. Bacterial biofilm: from the natural environment to infectious diseases. *Nat Rev Microbiol.* 2004;**2**(2):95–108.

Harrison-Balestra C, Cazzaniga AL, Davis SC, *et al.* A wound-isolated Pseudomonas aeruginosa grows a biofilm in vitro within 10 hours and is visualised by light microscopy. *Dermatol Surg.* 2003;**29**(6):631–635.

Hill KE, Davies CE, Wilson MJ, *et al.* Molecular analysis of the microflora in chronic venous leg ulceration. *J Med Microbiol.* 2003;**52**(4):365–369.

Hill KE, Malic S, McKee R, *et al.* An in vitro model of chronic wound biofilms to test wound dressings and assess antimicrobial susceptibilities. *J Antimicrob Chemother.* 2010;**65**(6):1195–1206.

James GA, Swogger E, Wolcott R, *et al.* Biofilms in chronic wounds. *Wound Repair Regen.* 2008;**16**(1):37–44.

Jeffersen K. What drives bacteria to produce a biofilm? *FEMS Microbiol Lett.* 2004;**236**(2):163–173.

Jensen PØ, Bjarnsholt T, Phipps R, *et al.* Rapid necrotic killing of polymorphonuclear leukocytes is caused by quorum sensing-controlled production of rhamnolipid by Pseudomonas aeruginosa. *Microbiology.* 2007;**153**(5):1329–1338.

Johansen C, Falholt P, Gram L. Enzymatic removal and disinfection of bacterial biofilms. *Appl Environ Microbiol.* 1997;**63**(9):3724–3728.

Kennedy P, Brammah S, Wills W. Burns, biofilm and a new appraisal of burn wound sepsis. *Burns.* 2010;**36**(1):49–56.

Kirketerp-Møller K, Jensen PØ, Fazli M, *et al.* Distribution, organization, and ecology of bacteria in chronic wounds. *J Clin Microbiol.* 2008;**46**(8):2717–2722.

Klausen M, Heydorn A, Ragas P, *et al.* Biofilm formation by Pseudomonas aeruginosa wild type, flagella and type IV pili mutants. *Mol Microbiol.* 2003;**48**(6):1511–1524.

Leake JL, Dowd SE, Wolcott RD, *et al.* Identification of yeasts in chronic wounds using new pathogen-detection technologies. *J Wound Care.* 2009;**18**(3):103–104, 106, 108.

Leid JG, Shirtliff ME, Costerton JW, *et al.* Human leukocytes adhere to, penetrate, and respond to Staphylococcus aureus biofilms. *Infect Immun.* 2002;**70**(11):6339–6345.

Maddocks SE, Lopez MS, Rowlands RS, *et al.* Manuka honey inhibits the development of Streptococcus pyogenes biofilms and causes reduced expression of two fibronectin binding proteins. *Microbiology.* 2012;**158**(3):781–790.

Malic S, Hill KE, Hayes A, *et al.* Detection and identification of specific bacteria in wound biofilms using peptide nucleic acid fluorescence *in situ* hybridization (PNS FISH). *Microbiology.* 2009;**155**(8):2603–2611.

Mast BA, Schultz GS. Interactions of cytokines, growth factors, and proteases in acute and chronic wounds. *Wound Repair Regen.* 1996;**4**(4):411–420.

Nakagami G, Morohoshi T, Ikeda T, *et al.* Contribution of quorum sensing to the virulence of Pseudomonas aeruginosa in pressure ulcer infections in rats. *Wound Repair Regen.* 2011;**19**(2):214–222.

Nakagami G, Sanada H, Sugama J, *et al.* Detection of Pseudomonas aeruginosa quorum sensing signals in an infected ischemic wound: an experimental study in rats. *Wound Repair Regen.* 2008;**16**(1):30–36.

Nemoto K, Hirota K, Murakami K, *et al.* Effect of varidase (streptodornase) on biofilm of Pseudomonas aeruginosa. *Chemotherapy.* 2003;**49**(3):121–125.

Neut D, Tijdens-Creusen EJA, Bulstra SK, *et al.* Biofilms in chronic diabetic foot ulcers-a study of 2 cases. *Acta Orthopaedica.* 2011;**82**(3):383–385.

Oates A, Bowling FL, Boulton AJ, *et al.* Molecular and culture-based assessment of the microbial diversity of diabetic chronic foot wounds and contralateral skin sites. *J Clin Microbiol.* 2012;**50**(7):2263–2271.

O'Toole G, Kaplan HB, Kolter R. Biofilm formation as microbial development. *Annu Rev Microbiol.* 2000;**54**:49–79.

Parsek MR, Singh PK. Bacterial biofilms: an emerging link to disease pathogenesis. *Annu Rev Microbiol.* 2003;**57**:677–701.

Percival SL, Bowler PG, Dolman J. Antimicrobial activity of silver-containing dressings on wound microorganisms using an in vitro biofilm model. *Int Wound J.* 2007;**4**(2):186–191.

Percival SL, Bowler PG, Woods EJ. Assessing the effect of an antimicrobial wound dressing on biofilms. *Wound Repair Regen.* 2008;**16**(1):52–57.

Potera C. Forging a link between biofilms and disease. *Science.* 1999;**283**(409):1837–1839.

Redkar R, Kalns J, Butler W, *et al.* Identification of bacteria from a non-healing diabetic foot ulcer wound by 16S rDNA sequencing. *Mol Cell Probes.* 2000;**14**(3): 163–169.

Rhoads DD, Wolcott RD, Sun Y, *et al.* Comparison of culture and molecular identification of bacteria in chronic wounds. *Int J Mol Sci.* 2012;**13**(3):2535–2550.

Rickard AH, Colacino KR, Manton KM, *et al.* Production of cell-cell signalling molecules by bacteria from human chronic wounds. *J Appl Microbiol.* 2010;**108**(5):1509–1522.

Rickard AH, Gilbert P, High NJ, *et al.* Bacterial coaggregation: an integral process in the development of multi-species biofilms. *Trends Microbiol.* 2003;**11**(2): 94–100.

Roberts AEL, Maddocks SE, Cooper RA. Manuka honey is bactericidal against Pseudomonas aeruginosa and results in differential expression of oprF and algD. *Microbiology.* 2012;**158**(13):3005–3013.

Sauer K, Camper AK, Ehrlich GD, *et al.* Pseudomonas aeruginosa displays multiple phenotypes during development as a biofilm. *J Bacteriol.* 2002;**184**(4):1140–1154.

Schierle CF, de la Garza M, Mustoe TA, *et al.* Staphylococcal biofilms impair wound healing by delaying reepithelialisation in a murine cutaneous wound model. *Wound Repair Regen.* 2009;**17**(3):354–359.

Secor PR, James GA, Fleckman P, *et al.* Staphylococcus aureus biofilm and planktonic cultures differentially impact gene expression, mapk phosphorylation, and cytokine production in human keratinocytes. *BMC Microbiol.* 2011;**11**:143.

Serralta VW, Harrison-Balestra C, Cazzaniga AL, et al. Lifestyles of bacteria in wounds: presence of biofilms? *Wounds.* 2001;**13**(1):29–34.

Spoering AL, Lewis K. Biofilms and planktonic cells of Pseudomonas aeruginosa have similar resistance to killing by antimicrobials. *J Bacteriol.* 2001;**183**(23): 6746–6751.

Stewart PS, Costerton JW. Antibiotic resistance of bacteria in biofilms. *Lancet.* 2001;**358**(9276):135–138.

Stoodley P, Sauer K, Davies DG, et al. Biofilms as complex differentiated communities. *Annu Rev Microbiol.* 2002;**56**:187–209.

Stoodley P, Wilson S, Hall-Stoodley L, et al. Growth and detachment of cell clusters from mature mixed species biofilms. *Appl Environ Microbiol.* 2001;**67**(12): 5608–5613.

Sutherland I. The biofilm matrix—an immobilized but dynamic environment. *Trends Microbiol.* 2001;**9**(5):222–227.

Tapininen T, Sormunen R, Kaijalainen T, et al. Ultrastructure of Streptococcus pneumoniae after exposure to xylitol. *J Antimicrob Chemother.* 2004;**54**(1): 225–228.

Thomsen TR, Aasholm MS, Rudkjøbing VB, et al. The bacteriology of chronic venous leg ulcer examined by culture independent molecular methods. *Wound Repair Regen.* 2010;**18**(1):38–49.

Trøstrup H, Thomsen K, Christophersen LJ, et al. Pseudomonas aeruginosa biofilm aggravates skin inflammatory response in BALB/c mice in a novel chronic wound model. *Wound Repair Regen.* 2013;**21**(2):292–299.

Wang R, Starkey M, Hazan R, et al. Honey's ability to counter bacterial infections arises from both bactericidal compounds and QS inhibition. *Front Microbiol.* 2012;**3**(article 144):1–8.

Weinberg ED. Suppression of bacterial biofilms by iron limitation. *Med Hypoth.* 22004;**63**(5):863–865.

Whitchurch CB, Tolker-Nielsen T, Ragas PC, et al. Extracellular DNA required for bacterial biofilm formation. *Science.* 2002;**295**(5559):1487.

Wolcott RD, Cox S. More effective cell-based therapy through biofilm suppression. *J Wound Care.* 2013;**22**(1):26–31.

Wolcott RD, Gontcharova V, Sun Y, et al. Bacterial diversity in surgical site infections: not just aerobic cocci any more. *J Wound Care.* 2009;**18**(8):317–323.

Wolcott RD, Rhoads DD. A study of biofilm-based management of subjects with critical limb ischemia. *J Wound Care.* 2008;**17**(4):145–155.

Wolcott RD, Rumbaugh KP, James GA, et al. Biofilm maturity studies indicate sharp debridement opens a time-dependent therapeutic window. *J Wound Care.* 2010;**19**(8):320–328.

Chapter 7

Antimicrobial agents used in wound care

Chris Roberts

Objectives

On completing this chapter you should have knowledge and understanding of:

1　The difference between groups of antimicrobial agents
2　The difference between bacteriostatic and bactericidal agents
3　Why different antimicrobial agents are used in different circumstances
4　The various methods available for testing susceptibility.

Introduction to antimicrobial agents used in wound care

Antimicrobial agents (antimicrobials) are of major importance in the treatment of a wide range of infectious diseases, including skin and soft tissue infections. There are hundreds of different types and their use can be very confusing because of their different modes of action and spectrum of activity. As antimicrobial resistance has developed, it is important that their use is fully understood, especially in wound care where many antimicrobial-resistant strains are isolated. This chapter will explain some fundamental differences between the various groups of antimicrobials and describe their appropriate use in wound care.

Background

There is a huge diversity of organisms that can delay wound healing and as a result, a wide variety of antimicrobials are used, some topically and some systemically. There are fundamental differences between antibiotics used in the systemic treatment of infection and antiseptics commonly used topically on wounds for cleansing and reducing organism numbers on the wound bed.

Antimicrobials

Antimicrobial is a general term for any compound with a direct action on microorganisms used for treatment or prevention of infection. Antimicrobials are inclusive of antibacterials (antibiotics), antivirals, antifungals, antiprotozoals, disinfectants, and antiseptics.

Antimicrobials can be divided into a number of categories that are defined as:

Antibiotics

An antibiotic is a natural substance obtained from certain fungi and bacteria that can inhibit the growth of bacteria. They have a specific target site within the bacterial cell and are widely used in the prevention and treatment of infectious diseases. Examples are beta lactams (penicillins, cephalosporins), aminoglycosides (gentamicin), and macrolides (erythromycin).

Antiviral agents

For most viral infections there is no specific treatment but there are a few effective antiviral drugs. They are usually virus specific. Examples are aciclovir (herpes virus), ganciclovir (CMV), and amantadine (influenza virus).

Antifungal agents

The number of antifungal agents is limited and they are more toxic than antibiotics. Many antifungal agents are used to treat skin infections caused by dermatophytes. Examples include azole compounds (e.g. ketoconazole for superficial mycoses), amphotericin B (aspergillosis), and flucytosine (systemic fungal infection).

Antiparasitic agents

A number of compounds are available that will kill parasites but tend to be divided into those that will kill protozoa (unicellular organisms) or helminths (those with a complex structure). All these compounds are toxic to the parasite but can also be toxic for humans. Examples include quinine (malaria) and piperazine (ascariasis).

 KEY POINT

- **Compounds** that are administered for systemic infectious disease usually aim at a specific target site within the microorganism which reduces the toxicity for the human host.

Disinfectants

A disinfectant has a broad-spectrum effect on all vegetative forms of micro-organisms, including spores, but is usually toxic to tissues. They are used for sterilizing surfaces, lavatories, and feeding bottles. Some, for example, hypochlorites, have been and still are being used in some areas of wound healing. Their main use is in wound cleansing.

 KEY POINT

- **Broad-spectrum compounds** show activity against a wide range of organisms, for example, bacteria, viruses, fungi, and parasites.

Antiseptics

An antiseptic is a compound that can be applied to living tissue/skin and which inhibits the growth of microorganisms. For practical purposes, anti-septics are routinely thought of as topical agents, for application to skin and mucous membranes.

Within the wound healing literature there is a high degree of confusion surrounding these definitions. This was recognized by Leaper (2006) who clarified the subject and his conclusions are incorporated into the definitions used here.

Bacteriostatic versus bactericidal activity of antimicrobial agents

Depending upon the mode of action of the antibacterial agent, the effect on the bacteria can be bacteriostatic (stops growth of the bacteria but they can recover if the antimicrobial is removed) or bactericidal (kills the bacterium irrevocably). Bacteriostatic agents prevent the bacterial population from in-creasing and allow the host defences to cope with the bacterial infection. However, a bactericidal agent does not rely on the host defences and kills the bacterium without help. This is important when assessing which antibiotic to choose for systemic treatment of an infection; however, it is a simplistic way of categorizing how an agent may affect the successful or unsuccessful progression of a wound towards healing and can be subject to debate. Clin-ical cure depends largely on host factors and laboratory tests can only pro-vide a rough prediction of bacterial eradication (Pankey and Sabath 2004). Therefore, when assessing data on antimicrobial efficacy in order to choose the appropriate therapeutic option for the patient, it is important to establish consistency in interpretation of evidence from the **bench to the bedside**.

Methods for testing antimicrobial agents

Minimal inhibitory concentration

Minimal inhibitory concentrations (MICs) and minimal bactericidal concentrations (MBCs) are the common methods used to determine susceptibility to an antimicrobial agent. MIC is a quantitative susceptibility test and is usually performed by making twofold dilutions of the antimicrobial agent in liquid culture medium in tubes, inoculating it with a standard number of microorganisms, and incubating it at 35–37°C for 24 hours. The concentration of antimicrobial agent that inhibits visible growth of the test microorganism in the broth is called the MIC (see Figure 7.1). Subcultures from clear tubes are made on a solid culture medium and re-incubated for an additional 24 hours to determine the MBC.

 DEFINITION

- **Minimal inhibitory concentrations (MICs)** are the lowest concentrations of antimicrobial agent needed to inhibit growth of the microorganism.
- **Minimal bactericidal concentrations (MBCs)** are the lowest concentrations of antimicrobial agent needed to kill the microorganism.

Interpretation of test results

In Figure 7.1, there is turbid growth in the control tube, 1 mg/L, and 2 mg/L—therefore the MIC is 4 mg/L. The clear tubes are subcultured onto solid agar and the last one showing 'No growth' is the MBC (in this example, 8 mg/L).

Factors affecting MIC/MBC

There are a number of factors that can affect MIC/MBC such as presence of organic matter (e.g. blood and serum), culture medium, diluents, and inoculum density; therefore MICs/MBCs are carried out using standard methodology, specifying conditions, so results can be compared and methodology is portable between laboratories (National Committee for Clinical Laboratory Standards 1999).

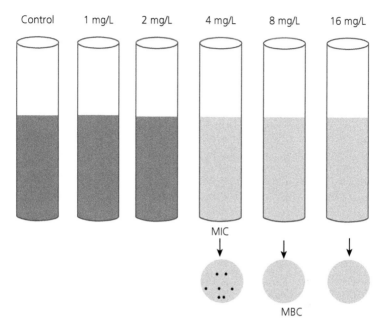

Figure 7.1 Diagram of the method for performing MICs.

The European Committee for Standardization (CEN) offers a number of protocols for evaluating antimicrobial agents (CEN 2006) and many are based on **in-use testing** (testing antimicrobial agents appropriate for their use) or **time-kill curves**. Here, a $\geq$ 99.9% decrease in the initial inoculum (which equates to a 3-$\log_{10}$ (1000-fold) reduction from the original inoculum size) in colony forming units is monitored over time and classed as satisfactory, especially for topical application (Peterson and Shanholtzer 1992). Some test procedures incorporate serum (actual or artificial) into the culture medium and the length of time the product is applied is taken into consideration to mimic realistic situations. For example, a wound cleanser would have to show a 3-log reduction in minutes because its application time will be minutes, whereas a dressing would have to show a 3-log reduction over a 24-hour period, to mimic the length of time it is in contact with the organisms.

Disc susceptibility testing

Typically antibiotic susceptibility testing is undertaken in clinical pathology laboratories using **disc susceptibility testing** where an antibiotic is impregnated into paper discs and placed on the surface of a sensitivity test agar seeded with the bacteria under test and incubated for 18 hours at 37°C (see Figure 7.2). The zone of inhibition (ZOI) is measured (diameter) (see Figure 7.3) and the bacterium is reported as sensitive or resistant to that antibiotic depending upon the size of the zone. These zone sizes have been calculated based on the standard methods used by all laboratories (the exact methodologies may differ between countries) and a number of factors are taken into account to ensure accuracy of reporting (Clinical and Laboratory Standards Institute 2012).

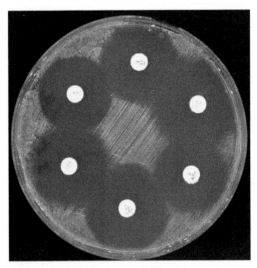

Figure 7.2 A typical antibiotic disc susceptibility test.

Reproduced by kind permission of Don Whitley Scientific Ltd. Copyright © 2015 Don Whitley Scientific Ltd., UK.

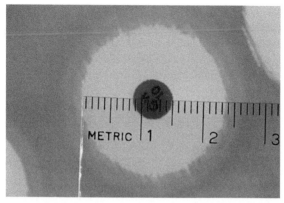

Figure 7.3 Measuring the zone of inhibition. The diameter is measured and compared to standard zone sizes for a particular antibiotic determined by the Clinical and Laboratory Standards Institute.

Reproduced from Centers for Disease Control and Prevention, Public Health Image Library (PHIL), Image ID# 10787, Gilda L. Jones, 1972, available from http://phil.cdc.gov/phil/details.asp?pid=10787.

Therapeutic monitoring

Antibiotic assays

Occasionally an antibiotic has to be used which can be highly toxic to the patient, leading to long-term conditions such as renal failure, deafness, and neurological disturbances. In order to prevent this from happening, these drugs are monitored by assessing the concentrations of the antimicrobial in patients' blood, urine, cerebrospinal fluid, and other bodily fluids prior to administration of each dose, ensuring levels are high enough to treat the infecting organism but low enough to prevent damage. Common antibiotics that are monitored are gentamicin and vancomycin.

Serum inhibitory titre

A serum sample taken from the patient during treatment is diluted and tested against the organism. The inhibitory titre is the lowest dilution of a serum that inhibits visible growth after incubation.

When should you stop using topical agents on wounds?

Best practice statements addressing the use of topical antiseptic/antimicrobial agents in wound management have agreed that if an antimicrobial agent is going to work then positive progress should be seen within the 10–14-day window after commencing treatment (Wounds UK 2011). This is not necessarily considered a time to stop treatment but a point when a holistic assessment of the patient and wound should be made to determine how to proceed. For example, if the wound is showing positive progress in terms of area reduction, quality of the wound bed, or a reduction in any signs and symptoms of infection, the following options could be considered: stop treatment or continue for another 2 weeks and reassess. If no progress is seen, choices regarding increasing dosage or changing frequency or selecting another antimicrobial should be made.

 KEY POINT

- Control microorganisms are used for every antimicrobial test undertaken in the laboratory to ensure standardization. An individual isolate is then tested from the patient. When reading publications reporting the efficacy of antimicrobial agents, it is important to note what control organisms are used and how many different strains have been tested.

- Definitions of MIC or MBC apply only to the particular organism (or even strain) against which it has been tested under the particular test conditions used.

- Some laboratory strains are particularly sensitive to agents such as silver, iodine, and so on and it is important to assess the relevance of the laboratory results to an antimicrobial's potential clinical performance.

- Many publications highlight positive findings in terms of an antimicrobial's ability to cause bacterial stasis or provide rapid kill in the laboratory, but it is important to look for evidence that the agent either kills bacteria in a wound or impacts on reducing infection rates. The former evidence can be reflected in quantitative measurements of total bacterial counts taken by swabs or tissue biopsy which is the gold standard. The latter evidence may present itself in either demonstrating a reduction in overall infection rates or relevant signs and symptoms of infection.

Systemic treatment strategies in wound care

Invasive wound infection needs systemic treatment with appropriate antibiotics. There are a large number of antibiotics available and they can be classified based on their mode of action. The available classes of antibiotics and a brief outline of how they work are detailed in Table 7.1.

Table 7.1 Different classes of antibiotics and their mode of action

Class of antibiotic	Mode of action	Bactericidal/ bacteriostatic
Beta lactams	**Bacterial cell wall synthesis**	Bactericidal
Penicillins, cephalosporins	Blocks cross-linking via competitive inhibition of transpeptidase enzyme	
Aminoglycosides	**Protein synthesis**	Bactericidal
Gentamicin, streptomycin	Irreversible binding to the 30s subunit of the bacterial ribosome	
Tetracyclines	**Protein synthesis**	Bacteriostatic
Tetracycline, minocycline	Blocks tRNA	
Macrolides	**Protein synthesis**	Bacteriostatic
Erythromycin, clarithromycin	Reversibly binds to 50s subunit of bacterial ribosome	
Chloramphenicol	**Protein synthesis**	Bacteriostatic
	Prevents protein chain elongation by inhibiting peptidyl transferase activity of the bacterial ribosome	
Lincosamide	**Protein synthesis**	Bacteriostatic
Clindamycin	Inhibits peptidyl transferase by interfering with aminoacyl tRNA complex	
Fluoroquinolones	**DNA synthesis**	Bactericidal
Nalidixic acid, ciprofloxacin, levofloxacin	Inhibits DNA gyrase enzyme which inhibits DNA synthesis	
Metronidazole	**DNA inhibition**	Bactericidal
	Metabolic by-products disrupt DNA	
Rifampicin	**Inhibits RNA transcription**	Bactericidal
	By inhibiting RNA polymerase	
Trimethoprim/sulphonamide	**Folic acid inhibition**	Bacteriostatic

Due to the increasing incidence of antibiotic resistance and the concern that drug-resistant strains may also become resistant to other antimicrobials including antiseptics used in wound care, it is very important that antimicrobial treatments are more regulated. This is especially true for administration of systemic antibiotics. There are antibiotic policies available within most healthcare settings that have been formulated by the infection control officer, the consultant microbiologist, and the pharmacist, in consultation with the various specialities. It is important that these policies are adhered to and unnecessary antibiotics are not prescribed as this may potentiate the problems of antimicrobial resistance even further. It is important that the local policies include appropriate antibiotic coverage for the common pathogens isolated within the hospital and community setting.

Types of topical antimicrobials

Silver

The antimicrobial properties of silver have been recognized since Roman times (silver ions leeching from silver coins were used to keep water microbiologically clean). It has a broad spectrum of activity against bacteria, yeasts, and fungi and has been used in modern-day wound healing since the early 1960s, when 0.5% silver nitrate aqueous solution was used as an alternative to antibiotics in the management of major burns. However, inactivation by protein and chloride in the wound meant application frequencies could be up to 15 times per day, to ensure sufficient levels were available to reduce the bacterial load. This created considerable pressure on staff to undertake dressing changes, in addition to staining seen on the patient and bedclothes. Silver linked to sulphadiazine carrier in a cream base (silver sulphadiazine) was introduced in the late 1960s and this reduced the frequency of application to once/twice daily as the levels of silver, through release and replenishment of ionic silver, were considerably improved (Gillett 1985). The cream base itself offered benefits with its soothing properties and ability to hold dressings in place whilst retention bandages were applied. Silver sulphadiazine cream was used in other clinical indications including chronic ulcers (Melotte et al. 1985).

Different forms of silver

Metallic silver is insoluble and therefore inactive as an antimicrobial. However, it is chemically reactive and forms a variety of silver salts. Four different states of silver exist: Ag^+, Ag^{++}, Ag^{+++}, and Ag^0. Singly charged silver, Ag^+, is the most biologically active. There are a number of different silver salts used in silver dressings—silver nitrate, silver sulphadiazine, silver acetate, and silver chloride—each with their own properties. In addition, nanocrystalline silver (Burrell 2003) is incorporated into dressings. This is produced by chemical reduction of silver and the resultant structure/shape of the nanoparticle in solution portrays different physical, biochemical, and antimicrobial properties. The average particle size of nanocrystalline silver is 20–120 nm when sputtered by vapour deposition onto a dressing surface, creating a larger surface area and more availability of silver ions. Continual sustained release of Ag$^+$ occurs when exposed to water, over 3–7 days from the Ag$^\circ$/Ag$^+$ complexes, and the reported levels remain at approximately 100 parts per million facilitating fewer dressing changes provided the dressing is kept moist and the exudate is managed effectively (Dunn and Edwards-Jones 2004). It is important to remember it is the structure and not the chemistry that dictates antimicrobial activity. All modern-day silver-containing products have an excellent safety profile and little evidence exists, if any, to show any delayed wound healing in clinical use.

 KEY POINT

- Numerous wound dressings containing various salts/states of silver at differing concentrations exist.

- The mechanism of release of silver is common between all dressings: through ionic exchange with chloride ions present in exudate, positively charged silver ions (Ag$^+$) are formed and become bioavailable.

- Quoted levels of silver vary considerably between manufacturers: from 1 ppm available silver for Aquacel Ag®, 20 ppm for Silvercel®, and 70–100 ppm for Acticoat™.

- Bioavailablity of silver ions is reduced in the presence of protein and chloride in exudate and final levels will be dictated by the release and replenishment profile (equilibrium will never be reached in a wound) which will vary from minute to minute depending on exudate output.

- In the literature, Edwards-Jones (2006) and Warriner and Burrell (2005) conclude that a level between 20 and 40 ppm ionic silver is required for clinical effectiveness but little support is supplied to validate these statements.

KEY POINT (continued)

♦ In terms of preventing the development of bacterial resistance, Chopra (2007) states: 'Dressings that release low levels of silver ions are likely to be more dangerous in terms of selection for resistance, especially if the silver ion concentration is sub-lethal. Faster acting dressings will inevitably present less risk because organisms are more likely to be killed, thereby eliminating possibilities for enrichment of the resistant population through growth and division, especially in the context of mutational development of resistance.'

♦ To date, in clinical practice, there has been no resistance development associated with the use of any modern-day silver dressing.

Iodine

Iodine is a highly effective antimicrobial that has been used in the treatment of wounds for over 150 years. It has a broad spectrum of activity and is effective against all bacterial species associated with wound infections and also a wide range of fungi, yeasts, protozoa, and viruses (Sibbald et al. 2011). However, it is reported to be painful on open wounds, irritates tissues, and can also cause allergic reactions. In addition, iodine stains the skin an intense yellow-brown colour, possesses an unpleasant odour, and is generally not stable in solution. In the early 1950s, iodophors (complexes of iodine and a solubilizing agent or carrier that increases solubility whilst sustaining release of iodine) were developed that retained the antimicrobial activity whilst removing the undesirable side effects. Iodine is carried in aggregates or micelles (lipid molecules that arrange themselves in a spherical form in aqueous solutions) which act as reservoirs of iodine. Once in contact with fluid the micelles slowly disperse, resulting in the controlled release of low concentrations of iodine. The activity is dependent on the amount of available iodine released from the iodophor. The two most commonly used iodophors in wound dressings are povidone iodine, a chemically bound complex between triiodide and povidone, and cadexomer iodide, an iodine and polysaccharide complex (Cooper 2007).

Cadexomer iodine

Cadexomer iodine consists of small, spherical, hydrophilic polysaccharide beads containing 0.9% iodine. In the presence of exudate, they absorb fluid and swell, allowing the slow and sustained release of iodine from the enlarged pores in the beads. The beads can absorb wound debris and help with cleansing the wound. Cadexomer iodine is available as a powder, dressing, or ointment and the most common adverse effects are a burning or stinging sensation on application, local irritation, redness, and eczema (Vermeulen et al. 2010).

 FACT

A number of studies have reported that cadexomer iodine can have a stimulatory effect on re-epithelialization of wounds; however, the mode of action is not clearly understood.

Inadine
Inadine is used for the management of suture lines and ulcerative wounds, including diabetic foot ulcers, for the prevention of infection in minor burns, and minor traumatic skin loss injuries, and in conjunction with systemic antibiotics in heavily infected wounds. The povidone iodine dressing, designed as a non-adherent wound-contact material, consists of a knitted viscose fabric impregnated with a polyethylene glycol (PEG) base containing 10% povidone iodine, equivalent to 1% available iodine, which is released in the presence of wound exudate. The water-soluble carrier, PEG, allows easy dressing removal but these dressings usually require daily application.

Iodine-based surgical scrub preparations also play a role in the prevention of surgical wound infections as skin disinfectants. These are used as an antiseptic for preoperative decontamination of the patient's skin at the site of a planned invasive procedure, and the hands of surgeons and theatre staff. The aim is to reduce skin flora and to prevent translocation into the underlying tissue by a scalpel or needle that may otherwise lead to infection of the wound. Surgical hand disinfection is carried out to remove transient and residential bacterial flora from the hands of the surgeon, to prevent contamination of the surgical site should the glove become punctured or damaged.

Polyhexamethylene biguanide
Polyhexamethylene biguanide (PHMB) is a heterodisperse (i.e. contains particles of varying sizes) mixture of polymers and has been used as an antiseptic and disinfectant for over 60 years. It has a broad spectrum of activity against bacteria, yeasts, and fungi. Due to its effective antimicrobial activity,

chemical stability, low toxicity, and reasonable cost, it has been widely used as swimming pool sanitizer, contact lens disinfectant, and more recently as an antimicrobial agent in modern wound management.

PHMB consists of positively charged molecules that attach and bind to the outer membrane of the negatively charged bacterial cell, causing areas of dysfunction and allowing PHMB to penetrate the inner membrane (Broxton et al. 1984). This causes the cell to lose control of normal transmembrane ion exchange, leading to increased fluidity, permeability, loss of integrity, and cell death. Similar effects are seen with the use of chlorhexidine. Studies indicate that PHMB does not interact with the neutral phospholipids in human cell membranes; however, it strongly interacts with the acidic lipids of bacterial cell membranes (Ikeda et al. 1984).

In clinical practice, commonly used concentrations of PHMB are 0.01%, 0.02%, or 0.04% available as antimicrobial irrigation solutions, cleansing gels, and dressings. Within the dressing formulations, there are products containing PHMB which provide an antimicrobial barrier, and dressing materials capable of donating PHMB to the wound surface (Bradbury and Fletcher 2011; Johnson and Leak 2011). In some products, PHMB is combined with a surfactant (betaine) which increases the cleansing activity and helps to remove biofilm.

Octenidine dihydrochloride

Octenidine dihydrochloride has two positively charged (cation) active centres in its molecule separated by a long aliphatic hydrocarbon chain (ten CH_2 groups). It binds readily to the negatively charged bacterial cell envelope, consequently disrupting the vital functions of the cell membrane and killing the cell. Data by Goroncy-Bermes (1998) show that the amount of the net negative charge of bacterial cell walls has an impact on the antimicrobial activity of cationic substances but does not prevent its penetration through the peptidoglycan layers or the damage to the cell membrane as demonstrated with octenidine. Octenidine dihydrochloride is used in wound cleansing solutions and gels at concentrations of 0.1% antiseptic. Solutions help to cleanse and loosen encrusted dressings when ready for changing. Water-based solutions also contain surfactant-like molecules such as ethylhexylglycerin which reduce the surface tension of the solution, enhancing its wetting behaviour.

Alternate forms of antibacterial agents

The wound infection consensus document launched in Toronto by the World Union of Wound Healing Societies (2008) refers to honey, tea tree oil, and maggots as an alternative compared to the more traditionally recognized antimicrobials.

Honey

The earliest record of the use of honey in wound treatment is noted on a fragment of a clay tablet dated to approximately 4500 years ago. Honey stopped being used in modern medicine in the 1970s and was re-introduced in the 1990s when a new generation of wound care products was developed. Molan et al. (1999) highlight a number of components of medical-grade honey that make it effective as an antimicrobial which include (1) its hygroscopic effect (meaning it draws moisture out of the environment) due to its high sugar content, (2) the presence of hydrogen peroxide, (3) the low pH (acidic— mean 4.4), and (4) the Unique Manuka Factor (UMF®) with its associated antibacterial peptides in some honeys. Most unprocessed honeys produce antimicrobial hydrogen peroxide by the activation of the enzyme glucose oxidase, which oxidizes glucose to gluconic acid and hydrogen peroxide. However, hydrogen peroxide can be degraded by an enzyme catalase, which can be found in wound fluid.

Manuka (*Leptospermum*) honey is made from nectar derived from a standard mixture of different *Leptospermum* spp. The *Leptosperum* spp. of plants are known by a number common names in Australia and New Zealand including Tea Tree, Manuka, Goo bush, and Jelly bush and at least 79 species have been described (Molan 2001). Unlike many common honeys, peroxide activity is **not** lost in the presence of catalase and it retains activity. They are also known as non-peroxide honeys because there are other unidentified components that contribute to the antimicrobial activity. A descriptor of UMF® has been given to these components. The number that follows the UMF®, for example, 10, means that the honey is 10 times more active than the standard antiseptic. The highest recorded level is around 20.

 DEFINITION

Catalase is an enzyme that degrades hydrogen peroxide and is found in wound fluid.

 KEY POINT

Honeys used for wound care should be medically certified honeys licensed as a medical product for professional wound care and not 'table honeys' that can be purchased over the counter as these may contain bacteria

The physical properties of honey play a part in its effectiveness as a wound dressing. Because of its viscosity, honey is claimed to provide a protective barrier which prevents cross infection. Also, because of its osmolarity drawing fluid out of the tissues it helps cleanse wounds providing a moist healing environment. This also means that dressings may not stick to the surface of wounds as they sit on a layer of diluted honey. There appears to be no growth of new tissue into the dressing so minimal pain on removal is claimed to be achieved.

As with many wound healing agents few randomized trials exist on the clinical efficacy of honey to complement the plethora of publications that demonstrate laboratory efficacy and successful case outcomes following its use and some randomized controlled trials found in the literature do not show significant benefits (Jull et al. 2008).

Larval therapy

There has been renewed interest in the use of maggots in wound healing. Larvae of the medicinal blow fly species (*Lucilia sericata*) have created a niche in therapeutic options called biosurgery. They are easy to culture in sterile conditions, have convenient life cycles, and are relatively hardy, withstanding the harsh environment of wounds that may also contain drugs. In particular, they avoid feeding on live tissue and can also be cooled for transport in sterilized containers and stored at 5°C (Wounds UK 2013). They are provided in special gauze bags that allow them to reach the tissue being treated. Antimicrobial enzymes are secreted which digest necrotic tissue and this is absorbed by the maggot, leaving the wound bed clean. More recently, a peptide known as lucifesin has been purified from larval secretions and exhibits a high degree of potency against wound pathogens (Jaklic et al. 2008).

Plants and plant oils

A wide variety of plants, their components flowers, fruits, leaves, grasses, roots, seeds, and herbs, demonstrate antimicrobial activity (Namita and Mukesh 2012). Essential oils from plants consist of a variety of hydrocarbons, and depending upon the ratios of major and minor components unique to a particular essential oil, contribute to the chemical composition. Tea tree oil is the most well-known essential oil from the leaves of the Australian *Melaleuca alternifolia* tree, a member of the botanical family *Myrtaceane*. The oil from the leaves is used medicinally and has found use in wound management. Scientific studies over recent years have shown it to be effective against bacterial, viral, and fungal organisms (Carson et al. 1998; Brady et al. 2006) whilst being a powerful immunostimulant, increasing the body's ability to fight off illness or infection. The potential exists for tea tree oil or combinations of this antiseptic with other aromatics to be used successfully in wound healing due to both good antibacterial and antiseptic activity and compatibility with dressing materials (Edwards-Jones et al. 2004). Palaniappan and Holley (2010) found that natural oils could increase antibiotic susceptibility of drug-resistant bacteria which may open up a new path to achieving success in winning the fight against the emergence of 'superbugs' being seen in wound healing and other clinical disciplines.

Conclusion

It is hoped that the reader will appreciate the challenges that present in determining appropriate antimicrobial treatment strategies for at-risk or infected wounds. The translation of laboratory values of both MICs and MBCs to clinical success lacks some certainty due to the complexities associated with both the patient and their wound. However, regular surveillance of progress at 7–14-day intervals will help gain confidence that the chosen antimicrobial is moving the wound forward from its stalled state. If there is no improvement, then decisions relating to changes in dose, frequency of application, or chosen antimicrobial can be made.

References

Bradbury S, Fletcher J. Prontosan® made easy. *Wounds Int.* 2011;**2**:1–6.

Brady A, Loughlin R, Gilpin D, *et al.* In vitro activity of tea-tree oil against clinical skin isolates of meticillin-resistant and -sensitive Staphylococcus aureus and coagulase-negative staphylococci growing planktonically and as biofilms. *J Med Microbiol.* 2006;**55**:1375–1380.

Broxton P, Woodcock P, Heatley F, *et al.* Interaction of some polyhexamethylene biguanides and membrane phospholipids in Escherichia coli. *J Appl Bacteriol.* 1984;**57**:115–124.

Burrell RE. A scientific perspective on the use of topical silver preparations. *Ostomy Wound Manage.* 2003;**49** Suppl 5:A19–24.

Carson CF, Riley TV, Cookson BD. Efficacy and safety of tea tree oil as a topical antimicrobial agent. *J Hosp Infect.* 1998;**40**;175–178.

European Committee for Standardization (CEN). *EN 14885 Chemical Disinfectants and Antiseptics—Application of European Standards for Chemical Disinfectants and Antiseptics.* Brussels: European Committee for Standardization; 2006.

Chopra I. The increasing use of silver based products as antimicrobial agents—a useful development or cause for concern. *J Antimicrob Chemotherapy.* 2007;**59**:587–590.

Clinical and Laboratory Standards Institute (CLSI). *Performance Standards for Antimicrobial Disk Susceptibility Tests; Approved Standard—Eleventh Edition.* Wayne, PA: Clinical and Laboratory Standards Institute: 2012. Available from: http://antimicrobianos.com.ar/ATB/wp-content/uploads/2012/11/01-CLSI-M02-A11-2012.pdf

Cooper RA. Iodine revisited. *Int Wound J*. 2007;**4**:124–137.

Dunn K, Edwards-Jones V. The role of Acticoat with nanocrystalline silver in the management of burns. *Burns*. 2004;**30** Suppl 1:S1–S9.

Edwards-Jones V. Antimicrobial and barrier effects of silver against methicillin-resistant Staphylococcus aureus. *J Wound Care*. 2006;**15**:285–290.

Edwards-Jones V, Buch R, Shawcross SG, et al. Effect of essential oils on Staphylococcus aureus using a dressing model. *Burns*. 2004;**30**:772–777.

Gillett AP. Antibiotic prophylaxis and therapy in burns. *J Hosp Inf*. 1985;**6** Suppl B:59–66.

Goroncy-Bermes P. Investigation into the efficacy of disinfectants against MRSA and VRE. *Zentralbl Hyg Umweltmed*. 1998;**201**:297–309.

Ikeda T, Ledwith A, Bamford CH, et al. Interaction of a polymeric biguanide biocide with phospholipid membranes. *Biochem Biophys Acta*. 1984;**769**:57–66.

Jaklic D, Lapangie A, Zupancic K, et al. Selective antimicrobial activity of maggots against pathogenic bacteria. *J Med Microbiol*. 2008;**57**:617–625.

Johnson S, Leak K. Evaluating a dressing impregnated with polyhexamethylene biguanide. *Wounds*. 2011;**7**:20–25.

Jull A, Walker N, Parag V, et al. Randomised control trial of honey-impregnated dressings for venous ulcers. *Br J Surg*. 2008;**95**:175–182.

Leaper DJ. Silver dressings—their role in wound management. *Int Wound J*. 2006;**3**:282–294.

Melotte P, Hendrix B, Mullie A, et al. Efficacy of 1% silver sulphadiazine cream in treating the bacteriological infections of leg ulcers. *Curr Ther Res*. 1985;**37**:197–202.

Molan PC. The role of honey in the management of wounds. *J Wound Care*. 1999;**8**:415–418.

Molan PC. Honey as a topical antibacterial agent for treatment of infected wounds. *World Wide Wounds*. 2001. Available from: http://www.worldwidewounds. com/2001/november/Molan/honey-as-topical-agent.html

Namita P, Mukesh R. Medicinal plants used as antimicrobial agents: a review. *Int Res J Pharm*. 2012;**3**:31–40.

National Committee for Clinical Laboratory Standards. *Methods for Determining Bactericidal Activity of Antimicrobial Agents; Approved Guideline, M26-A*. Wayne, PA: National Committee for Clinical Laboratory Standards; 1999.

Palaniappan K, Holley RA. Use of natural antimicrobials to increase antibiotic susceptibility of drug resistant bacteria. *Int J Food Microbiol*. 2010;**140**:164–168.

Pankey GA, Sabath LD. Clinical relevance of bacteriostatic versus bactericidal mechanisms of action in the treatment of Gram-positive infections. *Clin Infect Dis*. 2006;**38**:864–870.

Peterson LR, Shanholtz CJ. Tests for bactericidal effects of antimicrobial agents: technical performance and clinical relevance. *Am Soc Microbiol*. 1992;**5**:420–432.

Sibbald RG, Leaper DJ, Queen D. Iodine made easy. *Wounds Int*. 2011;**2**:s1–s6.

Vermeulen H, Westerbos SJ, Ubbink DT. Benefit and harm of iodine in wound care: a systematic review. *J Hosp Inf.* 2010;**76**:191–199.

Warriner R, Burrell RE. Infection and the chronic wound—a focus on silver. *Adv Skin Wound Care.* 2005;**18** Suppl 1:1–12.

World Union of Wound Healing Societies (WUWHS). *Principles of Best Practice: Wound Infection in Clinical Practice. An International Consensus.* London: MEP Ltd; 2008. Available from: http://www.mepltd.co.uk

Wounds UK. *Best Practice Statement: The Use of Topical Antiseptic/Antimicrobial Agents in Wound Management* (2nd ed). London: Wounds UK; 2011.

Wounds UK. *Larval Debridement Therapy. An Economic, Scientific and Clinical Evaluation.* London: Wounds UK; 2013.

Chapter 8

Dressings used in wound care

Madeleine Flanagan

Objectives

After completing this chapter you should have knowledge and understanding of:

1 The different types of dressings available in wound care
2 The principles of managing and treating critical colonization and wound infection
3 The importance of using wound bed preparation to develop a management protocol for infected wounds
4 How wound dressings can optimize local conditions at the wound bed to effectively manage symptoms associated with wound infection
5 How to identify the indications for use of topical antimicrobial wound dressings.

Introduction to dressings used in wound care

A wide variety of dressings are available for wound care practitioners and are used depending upon their function and the position, type, and severity of the wound. The main purpose of the dressing is to promote quick healing and to prevent further harm including infection. Dressings are made of sophisticated materials that can modulate the wound bed surface and provide the correct environment to facilitate wound healing. The various dressings can be classified depending upon their function and this will described in the chapter, with specific reference to their role in managing infection.

Background

Modern wound dressings are categorized on how they function. They include gauze, gels, hydrocolloids, foams, alginates, hydrogels, films, granules, and beads and are briefly described in Table 8.1.

Table 8.1 Modern wound dressings and their properties

Class of dressing	Function of the dressing
Hydrogels	Hydrogels contain > 80% water and are cohesive and remain on the wound. They facilitate debridement for dry fibrin and dry necrosis
Alginate–hydrofiber dressings	These are highly absorbent and are used for wet slough, necrosis, and heavily exuding wounds. These have excellent gelling properties and usually require a secondary dressing
Hydrocellular dressings	Hydrocellular dressings are absorbent, semi-permeable/waterproof dressings indicated for the treatment of low to moderately exuding wounds
Hydrocolloid dressings	Hydrocolloid is composed of carboxymethylcellulose and absorbs, swells, and gels. Hydrocolloid dressings are recommended for granulation and epithelialization phases (thin hydrocolloids)
Basic greasy dressings	These are composed of a loose mesh of cotton/viscose impregnated with a fatty substance and are used mainly in the epithelialization phase
Contact layers	Contact layers are composed of a tight mesh of a synthetic material coated with special compounds and are recommended for use at the end of the granulation and epithelialization phase
Active dressings	These dressings contain active substances, for specific purposes:
	To stimulate wound healing
	To provide an antibacterial action
	To control unpleasant odours
Carbon dressings	Carbon dressings are odour-absorbing

The ideal dressings should allow effective oxygen perfusion for the regenerating cells, may ease pain, absorb exudate, help with debridement, promote healing, protect from infection, and reduce stress for the patient. Irrespective of its function, the main aim of the dressing is to create an environment to facilitate moist wound healing (Winter 1962).

No single dressing is suitable for the management of all wound types and each phase of wound healing and the attributes of an ideal wound dressing are described in Table 8.2. Therefore the wound care practitioner must use the most appropriate dressing for the patient.

Table 8.2 Ideal properties of modern wound dressings

Property	Function
Fluid control	Ability to absorb wound exudate and to donate water to a dry wound
Low adherence	Trauma-free dressing removal
Physical barrier	Prevents bacterial contamination from the atmosphere and further damage to the tissue
Odour control	Prevents or minimizes wound odour
Microbial control	Bacteria need to be contained or removed
Debridement	Some dressings can accelerate the debridement process (i.e. removal of necrotic tissue) by providing the appropriate moisture, pH, and temperature
Haemostatic effect	Prevention of bleeding to prevent excessive blood loss (important in surgical or traumatic wounds)
Reduced scarring	Any dressing that can reduce scar formation is of great benefit
Metal ion metabolism	Some metal ions are important in cellular activity, e.g. inhibition or activation of enzymes

Source: data from Qin Y. Advanced wound dressings, *Journal of the Textile Institute*, Volume 92, Issue 2, pp.127–138, Copyright © 2001 Informa UK Ltd.

In addition, a full understanding of the type of wound being treated (i.e. acute or chronic), the phase of healing, and the patient's health must be known for effective wound management. The wound type (e.g. a deep burn wound) may necessitate the use of skin substitutes to provide a suitable wound bed for the re-epithelialization process to allow closure. An acute surgical site with sutures may just need an adhesive film to allow the wound to be inspected for signs of infection without removal, provide sufficient moisture for rapid healing, and act as a barrier to prevent infection. In a chronic non-healing wound, wound dressings are used in the preparation of a healthy wound bed and also to accelerate the endogenous healing process.

Apparent wound infection may occur at any stage of the healing process and with appropriate treatment should resolve without too many problems. If left untreated or if a wound fails to respond to treatment, an infected wound can lead to systemic disease and may be fatal. An alternative consequence can be delayed wound closure or the development of a chronic non-healing wound due to an imbalance of endogenous host factors and exogenous bacterial factors. These cause an imbalance of the production and degradation of the extracellular matrix of the wound bed. The loss of skin integrity and exposure of underlying tissue provides a moist, warm micro-environment that encourages bacterial multiplication and proliferation. The type and abundance of microorganisms in a wound depends on location, depth, oxygen supply, host factors, and tissue perfusion (Dowd et al. 2008; Bjarnsholt et al. 2008; James et al. 2008). Judicious selection of wound dressings can help to optimize local environmental conditions at the wound bed to stimulate healing.

Although many dressing products have been established for a long time, there are comparatively few large, well-randomized studies to support their use (Thomas 2010). Most of the evidence for their use is generated through product evaluation and detailed case studies. This is especially the case for the use of dressings impregnated with topical anti-microbial agents where systematic reviews have not demonstrated the efficacy of one topical antimicrobial over another as the published data consist of small, poor quality studies where dressings were used for ex-tended periods (Vermeulen et al. 2007; Brölmann et al. 2012).

Wound bed preparation

Before wound closure occurs, physiological barriers to healing must be eliminated so that the local wound environment can support the delicate process of tissue repair. This requires the removal of non-viable tissue, con-trol of bacterial burden, maintenance of moisture balance, and provision of an environment to promote epithelialization for each patient (Falanga 2000; Schultz et al. 2003) following careful patient assessment (Sibbald et al. 2000). WBP provides a framework for clinical decision-making so that non-healing wounds can be identified early and advanced interven-tions implemented. Wounds that fail to respond to standard moist wound dressings should be carefully reassessed for signs and symptoms that the bacteria colonizing the wound (wound bioburden) may be delaying heal-ing and stepped up to topical antimicrobial dressings. Figure 8.1 shows a typical non-healing venous ulcer with high bioburden, necrotic tissue, and copious exudate and Figure 8.2 shows the relationship between bioburden and the types of dressing selection. The step wise approach of WBP helps ensure that antimicrobial dressings are targeted at individuals with critic-ally colonized or locally infected wounds. Early intervention maximizes the chance of successful treatment without having to use systemic antibiot-ics. The rationale for dressing choice is often guided by local wound man-agement policies, or guidelines and many excellent examples are available on the Internet.

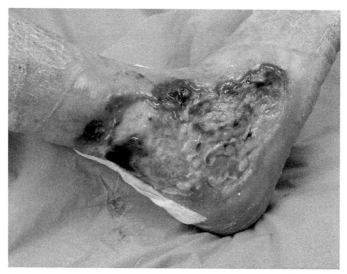

Figure 8.1 A non-healing venous ulcer: high bioburden, necrotic tissue, and copious exudate.

Dressing infected wounds

 KEY POINT

Selection of a dressing for an infected wound is to create optimal local conditions at the wound bed to manage symptoms associated with cutaneous infection to limit progression from localized colonization to invasive/deep tissue infection. Many wound dressings are selected based on personal expert opinion as the quality of evidence to support the use of one wound dressing over another is limited (Brölmann et al. 2012). Selection is based upon:

- Controlling bacterial burden
- Reducing necrotic burden
- Regulating moisture balance
- Controlling wound odour
- Preventing the spread of infection
- Protecting the wound and surrounding skin.

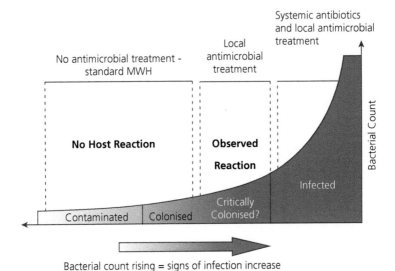

Bacterial count rising = signs of infection increase

Figure 8.2 Relationship between bioburden and dressing selection. Bacterial colonization is of no clinical significance and should not be confused with wound infection. A recognized definition of wound infection is if a wound contains at least 10^6 bacteria/g of tissue. But this only counts bacterial dose and does not consider other variables. So some chronic wounds may contain 10^8 bacteria/g without any obvious signs of infection (host reactions).

Reproduced with permission from Edwards-Jones V. and Flanagan M. (2013) Wound infection. In: Flanagan M. (Ed.) *Wound Healing and Skin Integrity: Principles and Practice*. Chichester, UK: Wiley-Blackwell. Copyright © 2013 John Wiley and Sons, Ltd., UK.

Symptom management

Surgical site or an acute wound infection is often easy to clinically diagnose because the classic signs and symptoms are present. Diagnosis may be more complicated in a burn wound where there is a massive amount of inflammation because of the injury itself. However, individuals with chronic wounds frequently have compromised immune systems which can mean that they may not display classic signs of infection as they may not always elicit a host response. Instead, a sudden increase in wound symptoms, such as pain, exudate, and malodour, may be the first indicators of wound infection (Gardner et al. 2001) and if these symptoms appear then the symptoms will influence the dressing choice. The characteristics for identifying wound infection are summarized elsewhere in Chapter 4.

Controlling bioburden: dressings for wound debridement

Studies have demonstrated that as wounds heal, bacterial numbers start to fall (Trengove et al. 2000). Therefore it is important that the surface of wounds should be cleaned to ensure that organic matter such as pus, slough, extracellular products, biofilm, and exudate are removed as they are the ideal growth mediums for microorganisms (Edwards-Jones and Flanagan 2013). In addition, there is increasing evidence that wound debridement is one of the most effective methods of reducing bioburden as it helps to remove loosely adherent microorganisms and cellular debris (Wolcott et al. 2009). Studies have shown that there is a brief period immediately after wound debridement when microorganism numbers are reduced and the biofilm is disrupted. At this point, the application of a topical antimicrobial dressing may help stimulate wound healing (Wolcott et al. 2009). These local measures may be sufficient to reduce the bioburden sufficiently to allow healing to resume without the need for systemic antibiotic therapy. However, it must be remembered that debridement cannot remove all biofilm, so after a few days, local conditions may have deteriorated to allow the remaining biofilm to redevelop. As is often the case in wound management, there is limited evidence to support selection of one particular method of wound debridement over another and choice needs to consider individual assessment of the patient and wound (Figure 8.3).

Dressings for autolytic debridement

Autolytic debridement can be facilitated at the bedside using semi-occlusive dressings such as film dressings plus dressings with a high water content such as hydrogels, hydrocolloids, honey, and cadexomer iodine dressings (Sibbald et al. 2011). **Hydrogels** (available as flat sheets or amorphous gels) create a moist wound interface which enhances the activity of endogenous proteolytic enzymes within the wound, liquefying and separating necrotic tissue from healthy tissue. They effectively remove soft slough or firmer, more adherent dry eschar from the wound surface and are easy to apply. This technique is particularly useful if, for technical or medical reasons, more invasive procedures are not suitable for the patient.

Dressings for enzymatic debridement

Enzymatic agents have decreased in popularity as they are more difficult to use than other dressings. These products are topical formulations—gels, creams, and pastes that are derived from either proteolytic enzymes extracted from bovine plasma or pancreas, and fruit and plants such as papain from papaya, or bromelain from pineapple, or bacterial collagenase derived from

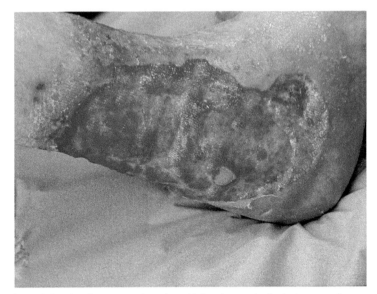

Figure 8.3 A healing venous leg ulcer: bioburden controlled, absence of necrotic tissue, and moisture balance regulated.

Clostridium histolyticum. These exogenous enzyme preparations are applied to the wound bed and are recommended if a hard, dry eschar is present. Enzymatic preparations are usually applied to the eschar edge, encouraging it to separate from the granulation tissue, but penetration of thick, necrotic tissue can be slow and may require crosshatching with a scalpel which needs to be performed by competent clinicians.

Dressings for biosurgical debridement

The use of sterile fly larvae in the treatment of sloughy, infected wounds is becoming more popular as larvae secretions contain chemicals with antimicrobial properties, which may help to increase wound pH which inhibits bacterial growth (Davydov 2011). The sheep blowfly larvae *Lucilia sericata* (Diptera: Calliphoridae) are applied as a dressing (usually they are encased in a loose meshed bag) and are used as they secrete collagenase and trypsin which liquefies necrotic tissue which is then ingested along with any microorganisms. The *Lucilia sericata* maggot is effective against a wide range of bacteria including *Clostridium perfringens*, meticillin-resistant *Staphylococcus aureus* (MRSA), and *Pseudomonas* spp. Contraindications include bleeding wounds, due to risk of blood vessel erosion, or highly exudating wounds, as larvae can drown.

Dressings for mechanical debridement

Mechanical debridement physically removes devitalized tissue from the wound bed and traditionally includes the use of wet-to-dry gauze dressings which is traumatic and painful but is still common in some clinical environments. Wet-to-dry gauze uses saline-soaked gauze which is allowed to dry and adhere to the wound surface. When removed, it mechanically disrupts the tissue at the wound surface and as it does not discriminate between devitalized necrotic tissue and healthy granulation tissue, this causes trauma.

An alternative approach to traditional mechanical debridement is the use of a disposable monofilament fibre pad that is moistened and gently rubbed across the wound bed in a circular motion to physically dislodge debris and slough from the wound surface. Clinicians can control the amount of tissue removed and stop if the patient experiences any discomfort. This method of debridement is becoming popular as it is quick, safe, inexpensive, and easy to use.

Controlling bacterial burden: antimicrobial dressings

One of the commonest methods of reducing bioburden in a critically colonized or infected wound is to apply topical antimicrobial dressings. Newer generation slow-release antimicrobial dressings enable control of resistant microbial species such as MRSA and vancomycin-resistant enterococci and have low toxicity and are less likely to induce resistance than antibiotics (Parsons 2005).

 KEY POINT

Recent best practice statements recommend that antimicrobial dressings should be checked daily and progress formally reviewed at 7 days and again a week later to evaluate treatment efficacy (Wounds International 2013). If after 2 weeks there is no wound improvement, then the dressing should be reviewed and consideration given to changing to one containing a different antimicrobial agent and the use of a systemic antibiotic. If there is wound improvement but with continuing signs of infection, then application of the same dressing should be continued. If there is wound improvement with no signs or symptoms of infection, then the antimicrobial dressing should be replaced by an appropriate non-antimicrobial dressing.

Chapter 7 details the antimicrobial agents used in wound care and they are incorporated into a variety of dressings. The physical properties of the dressing must not be compromised and wherever possible must release the antimicrobial agent slowly or effect a targeted release. The dressings should also show activity against microorganisms typically isolated from wounds namely *Staphylococcus aureus* (including MRSA), *Pseudomonas aeruginosa*, group A and C streptococci, *Escherichia coli, Klebsiella* spp., anaerobic bacteria, and yeasts including *Candida albicans*. The antimicrobial agents in the dressing should not be inactivated readily by organic matter found in the wound. Antimicrobial dressings are increasing in demand and popularity and are available with incorporated antimicrobials such as silver compounds, iodine, chlorhexidine, polyhexamethylene biguanide, or honey.

An alternative method for removal of microorganisms without using an antimicrobial agent is by their physical removal. Dressings coated with dialkylcarbamoyl chloride form a wound contact layer which irreversibly binds to bacteria and fungi which are removed along with the dressing at the point of dressing removal. These dressings are available as absorbent pads and packing materials, foams, and hydropolymer gels and absorb wound fluid, debride moist, sloughy wounds, and can also be used prophylactically to treat patients at high risk of wound infection.

Dressings for exudating wounds (regulation of moisture balance)

Increased exudate production associated with wound infection and heavy bioburden is one of the most difficult aspects to manage as a balance between exudate absorption or containment, maintenance of a moist wound environment, prevention of dressing adherence, and wound desiccation (drying out) is required. One of the most important considerations when selecting a dressing for a highly exuding wound is to establish the type, viscosity, and volume of wound fluid being produced as dressing choice is dependent on its absorbent capacity. They range from simple absorbent dressings which retain fluid until pressure is applied to newer superabsorbent cellulose and polymer dressings with advanced fluid retention properties allowing for extended wear time. The most commonly used dressings with absorptive properties are alginate, hydrofiber, foams, and those with hydroconductive properties.

Alginate

Alginate dressings are derived from sodium/calcium salts of alginic acid, obtained from seaweed (Thomas 2010). On contact with wound fluid, sodium salts in wound exudate exchange with the calcium in the alginate dressing to from a soft hydrophilic gel which maintains a moist environment at the wound surface. Alginate dressings are highly absorbent, promote autolytic debridement in moist wounds, lower the bioburden, and absorb proteinases (Sweeney et al. 2014). They can be combined with silver to increase antimicrobial activity and charcoal to reduce odour and are conformable, making them useful in irregular-shaped infected wounds and sinus.

Hydrofiber

Hydrofiber dressings are composed of sodium carboxymethylcellulose which absorbs wound fluid and transforms into a soft gel. Hydrofiber and alginate dressings are sometimes confused as they look similar, share the same clinical indications (sloughy, infected, and highly exudating wounds), and have similar performance characteristics.

Polyurethane foam dressings

Polyurethane foam dressings are also popular for management of infected wounds as they are highly absorbent with low adherence. Most have an outer semipermeable membrane that allows fluid to pass into the foam to minimize maceration of the surrounding skin and are easy to use (Thomas 2010).

Wound dressings have always been the first-line management option for controlling moisture balance in wounds although new technologies offer the clinician a variety of alternatives e.g.:

Negative pressure wound therapy
The use of indirect fluid handling modalities such as compression therapy, wound drainage devices, and use of barrier products to protect the skin are an important adjunct to absorbent wound dressings.

Dressings for malodorous wounds

Infected wounds often have an offensive odour that can have a profound effect on patients and their families. Patients become embarrassed by smell and leakage from saturated dressings which can lead to social isolation, especially in chronic wounds that repeatedly become infected such as venous leg ulcers and fungating wounds. Malodour is a by-product of bacterial activity in hypoxic, devitalized tissue in the wound bed. In chronic wounds, anaerobic bacteria of the *Bacteroides* and *Clostridium* spp. are typically involved. Aerobic bacterial species, such as *Proteus*, *Klebsiella*, and *Pseudomonas* spp., may also be present but tend to produce less toxic by-products. Dressings containing topical antimicrobial agents can be an effective method of controlling wound odour, if other symptoms suggest their use; however they can be costly.

Activated charcoal dressings

Activated charcoal dressings are commonly used to contain wound malodour. These dressings usually contain a layer of charcoal cloth that attracts and binds the molecules responsible for wound odour. Activated charcoal dressings are available as a simple secondary cloth dressing or may incorporate other dressing materials, such as foam, alginate, or hydrofiber. In general, activated charcoal dressings work best when kept dry and when a complete seal is maintained over the wound by the dressing which is not always possible. The use of medical-grade honey (and honey dressings) can control wound odour as it is bactericidal and facilitates wound debridement. Essential oils can help disguise odour (Mercier and Knevitt 2005) as well as standard nursing interventions such as daily dressing changes and effective disposal of soiled dressings.

Dressings to alleviate wound pain

Wound pain is one of the most reliable symptoms of wound infection and usually occurs before any clinical signs of infection are evident (Gardner et al. 2001). The inflammatory response stimulated by invading microorganisms is the underlying cause of wound pain. The release of inflammatory mediators in infected wounds results in oedema and tissue damage which causes peripheral pain receptors to produce pain of increasing intensity, often described as a tender or intense, throbbing pain. Treatment aimed at reducing the bacterial burden of the wound should alleviate infection-related wound pain; therefore the use of broad-spectrum antimicrobial dressings and anti-inflammatory analgesia can be effective.

Wound care procedures may contribute to wound pain, for example, debridement, inappropriate cleansing technique, or use of dressings that adhere to the wound bed. Appropriate wound care practices include gentle cleansing by irrigation and using non-adherent dressings. Less frequent dressing changes will also help by reducing the need for painful wound care episodes.

Conclusion

A balance is needed when changing dressings on infected wounds, too frequent removal may not let topical antimicrobial agents have a lasting effect and may cause wound pain, whilst infrequent dressing change can cause dressings to become saturated and leak. This increases the risk of cross-infection and may cause wound deterioration. Dressing materials vary greatly in their fluid handling capacity so it is important to understand how different dressing materials function in order to make an appropriate choice. In infected wounds, they should be inspected daily to ensure they are intact, with no strikethrough and are not leaking. **Strict aseptic techniques** need to be used when changing and disposing of dressing and meticulous attention paid to hand washing techniques to avoid cross-contamination.

If dressings are unable to contain wound exudate from infected wounds, leakage occurs and the skin around the wound becomes soaked in chronic wound fluid which is rich in irritant proteases and pro-inflammatory cytokines (Trengove et al. 1999). The skin around infected wounds is at increased risk of breakdown due to maceration and the corrosive effects of proteolytic exudate. Skin protectants aim to prevent skin breakdown by protecting vulnerable skin from irritants and excess moisture. The introduction of synthetic barrier products which leave a thin protective layer on the skin has proven useful. Skin care systems are now available that provide a combination of products including liquid barrier films, moisturizing skin cleansers, and skin protectant creams.

Technological advances now offer clinicians a bewildering choice of dressings for infected wounds that sometimes leads to ineffective decision-making. There are a number of international clinical guidelines that demonstrate consensus on the principles of managing infected wounds and are accessible via the Internet (World Union of Wound Healing Societies 2008; Wounds International 2013; Wounds UK 2013).

 KEY POINT

How can I make sure that I am using antimicrobial dressings effectively?

The principles of using an antimicrobial dressing are:

- ◆ Conduct a thorough patient and wound assessment before deciding if an antimicrobial dressing is appropriate.
- ◆ Document the rationale for using an antimicrobial dressing in the patient's healthcare records
- ◆ Choose an antimicrobial dressing on the basis of patient and wound needs, for example, exudate level, wound depth, and odour control.
- ◆ Review treatment progress at 7 days and again at 14 days.
- ◆ Continued use of antimicrobial dressings after 14 days should be a team decision based on a review of current treatment objectives.

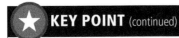

KEY POINT (continued)

- Antimicrobial dressings should be used in the context of a wound management protocol such as WBP.
- Manufacturers' instructions regarding indications, contraindications, and application methods must be followed at all times.

Source: data from International consensus, *Appropriate use of silver dressings in wounds: an expert working group consensus*. London: Wounds International, http://www.woundsinternational.com/media/issues/567/files/content_10381.pdf, accessed 01 Apr. 2015, Copyright © 2012 Wounds International, UK.

Further reading

European Wound Management Association (EWMA). EWMA document. Antimicrobials and non-healing wounds: Evidence, controversies and suggestions. *J Wound Care.* 2013;**22**(Suppl 5):S1–S89.

World Union of Wound Healing Societies. *Principles of Best Practice: Wound Infection in Clinical Practice. An International Consensus.* London: MEP Ltd; 2008. Available from: http://www.woundsinternational.com/clinical-guidelines/wound-infection-in-clinical-practice-an-international-consensus

References

Bjarnsholt T, Kirketerp-Møller K, Jensen PØ, *et al.* Why chronic wounds will not heal: a novel hypothesis. *Wound Repair Regen.* 2008;**16**:2–10.

Brölmann FE, Ubbink DT, Nelson EA, *et al.* Evidence-based decisions for local and systemic wound care. *Br J Surg.* 2012;**99**(9):1172–1183.

Davydov L. Maggot therapy in wound management in modern era and a review of published literature. *J Pharm Pract.* 2011;**24**(1):89–93.

Dowd SE, Sun Y, Secor PR, *et al.* Survey of bacterial diversity in chronic wounds using pyrosequencing, DGGE, and full ribosome shotgun sequencing. *BMC Microbiol.* 2008;**8**:43.

Edwards-Jones V, Flanagan M. Wound infection. In Flanagan M (ed) *Wound Healing and Skin Integrity Principles & Practice.* Wiley-Blackwell; 2013: 87–101.

European Wound Management Association (EWMA) EWMA document. Antimicrobials and non-healing wounds: Evidence, controversies and suggestions. *J Wound Care.* 2013;**22**(Suppl 5):S1–S89.

Falanga V. Classifications for wound bed preparation and stimulation of chronic wounds. *Wound Rep Regen.* 2000;**8**:347–352.

Gardner SE, Frantz, RA, Doebbeling B. The validity of the clinical signs and symptoms used to identify localized chronic wound infection. *Wound Repair Regen.* 2001;9:178–186.

James GA, Swogger E, Wolcott R, *et al.* Biofilms in chronic wounds. *Wound Repair Regen.* 2008;16:37–44.

Mercier D, Knevitt D. Using topical aromatherapy for the management of fungating wounds in a palliative care unit. *J Wound Care.* 2005;14:497–503.

Parsons D, Bowler PG, Myles V, *et al.* Silver antimicrobial dressings in wound management: a comparison of antibacterial, physical, and chemical characteristics. Wounds. 2005;17(8):222–232.

Qin Y. Advanced wound dressings. *J Textile Inst.* 2001;92:127–138.

Schultz G, Sibbald R, Falanga V, *et al.* Wound bed preparation: a systematic approach to wound management. *Wound Repair Regen Suppl.* 2003;11(2S):S1–S28.

Sibbald RG, Leaper DJ, Queen D. Iodine made easy. *Wounds Int.* 2011;2(2):S1–S6.

Sibbald RG, Williamson D, Orsted HL, *et al.* Preparing the wound bed—debridement, bacterial balance and moisture balance. *Ostomy Wound Manage.* 2000;46(11):14–35.

Sweeney IR, Miraftab M, Collyer G. A critical review of modern and emerging absorbent dressings used to treat exuding wounds. *Int Wound J.* 2012;9(6):601–612.

Thomas S. *Surgical Dressings and Wound Management.* Cardiff: Medetec Publications; 2010.

Trengove NJ, Bielefeldt-Ohmann H, Stacey MC. Mitogenic activity and cytokine levels in non-healing and healing chronic leg ulcers. *Wound Repair Regen.* 2000;8:13–25.

Trengove NJ, Stacey MC, Macauley S, *et al.* Analysis of the acute and chronic wound environments: the role of proteases and their inhibitors. *Wound Repair Regen.* 1999;7:442–452.

Vermeulen H, van Hattem JM, Storm-Versloot MN, *et al.* Topical silver for treating infected wounds. *Cochrane Database Syst Rev.* 2007;24(1):CD005486.

Winter G. Formation of the scab and the rate of epithelisation of superficial wounds in the skin of the young domestic pig. *Nature.* 1962;193:293–294.

Wolcott RD, Kennedy JP, Dowd SE. Regular debridement is the main tool for maintaining a healthy wound bed in most chronic wounds. *J Wound Care.* 2009;18(2):54–56.

World Union of Wound Healing Societies (WUWHS). *Principles of Best Practice: Wound Infection in Clinical Practice. An International Consensus.* London: MEP Ltd, 2008.

Wounds International. *International Consensus: Appropriate Use of Silver Dressings in Wounds.* London: Wounds International; 2013. Available from: http://www.woundsinternational.com/pdf/ content_10381.pdf

Wounds UK. *Best Practice Statement. The Use of Tropical Antimicrobial Agents in Wound Management* (3rd ed). London: Wounds UK; 2013.

Chapter 9

Infection prevention and control

Martin Kiernan

Objectives

On completing this chapter you should have knowledge and understanding of:

1 Healthcare-associated infections
2 Infection control policies associated with wound management
3 Prevention of infection
4 Common transmission and spread of infection.

Introduction to infection prevention and control

A patient with a wound (whether acute or chronic) is at risk of acquiring an infection during their course of treatment within a healthcare environment and this may be from their own skin (endogenous) or from the healthcare environment or staff (exogenous). The consequence of infection can create problems for the patient and need to be avoided wherever possible. Infection control has to be a priority for the patient and the wound care specialist in order to prevent infection whenever possible and manage other associated risks. This chapter will highlight the problems associated with wound infection and healthcare-associated infections (HCAIs).

Healthcare-associated infections

HCAIs are infections that are acquired after an individual has any form of interaction with healthcare. This is different from the former term of hospital-acquired infection (HAI) and is reflective of the change in the way that healthcare is delivered in locations outside of hospitals. Wounds that fall into this category may be acute (trauma or surgical) or chronic (pressure or leg ulcer) in nature. Thus a HCAI may occur in a new surgical wound or in a chronic wound that has been affected by cross-infection due to suboptimal practice of those caring for the wound.

The role of the wound in HCAI

Wounds are significant in HCAI in two ways. Firstly, a wound is a breach in skin integrity that enables microorganisms to colonize a wound and cause infection in the individual. Secondly the colonization of a wound with potential pathogens, even if not causing infection, serves as a reservoir for potential onward transmission. This is particularly significant when colonized with meticillin-resistant *Staphylococcus aureus* (MRSA) or multidrug-resistant Gram-negative bacteria. The colonized wound then becomes a risk to others in terms of potential transmission in addition to being a risk to the individual themselves should they have invasive medical devices present, for example, intravenous access lines or urinary catheters.

One study has examined the risk of wound carriage of multiresistant organisms and bloodstream infections and has reported a significant risk. In this work, 145 patients with a greater than stage 2 pressure sore were investigated (Braga et al. 2013). Over 75% had wounds that were colonized or infected with bacteria. *Staphylococcus aureus* was the largest group (21%), followed by Gram-negative bacteria. Sixty-five per cent were classed as multidrug-resistant organisms (MDROs) and these organisms were considered to be implicated in 54% of 56 bacteraemia episodes. The authors concluded that patients with a pressure ulcer, especially when colonized with MDROs, constitute a high-risk population for bacteraemia with a poor outcome.

The risks of transmission should also be considered and there is an increasing awareness of the role of the environment (Otter et al. 2011). There is also some evidence that organisms infecting wounds can contaminate the environment (Ray et al. 2010), probably via the vector of hands, and so the environment becomes a reservoir for onward transmission of pathogens (Boyce et al. 1997). In one study, *Streptococcus pyogenes* (Group A Strep) causing infection in a tracheostomy wound was found to have contaminated a third of patient curtains on the ward, resulting in two further patients and a staff member becoming infected (Mahida et al. 2014).

The techniques used within wound management can also have a deleterious effect on transmission of microorganisms. Debridement of the wound bed through the use of water jets is clinically effective; however, it is important that these procedures are carried out in a suitable environment since there is some evidence that considerable contamination of the environment can occur during this procedure (Sönnergren et al. 2013).

Current problems including costs of management

The wound infections most commonly associated with HCAI are those arising from surgical wounds. The human and financial cost of this is significant and in the most recent national prevalence survey, surgical site infections (SSIs) were the third highest HCAI (Health Protection Agency 2012).

 FACT

Reported HCAIs from the 2011 National Prevalence of Healthcare-associated Infections (England) are:

♦ Pneumonia and other respiratory infections: 22.8%

♦ Urinary tract infections: 17.2%

♦ Surgical site infections: 15.7%

♦ Clinical sepsis: 10.5%

♦ Gastrointestinal infections: 8.8%

♦ Bloodstream infections: 7.3%.

Given the ever-shortening postoperative length of stay, this is a significant level of infection. Data from national surveillance do not reflect the true burden of infection due to data collection being limited to inpatient and re-admission infections only. In 2010/2011 the national rate of infection for large bowel surgery was 10.1% (Health Protection Agency 2011), whereas surveillance carried out for the purposes of research in which more resources are given for case-finding with robust post-discharge surveillance demonstrated that the true rate was closer to 27%, nearly three times the national rate (Tanner et al. 2009). This important study also undertook a costing exercise in order to determine the financial burden of these infections. The additional cost of treating these patients was calculated to be £10,523, with 15% of these costs being borne by primary care. The two highest costs were incurred by extended length of stay and visits by district nurses as infected patients received an average of 19 visits at a cost of £64 per hour. The total annual cost of infection in one procedure in one hospital was estimated to be in excess of £720,000, with over £100,000 borne by primary care. Other studies estimate the cost of a SSI to be double that of an episode with no infection (Broex et al. 2009). One must also not forget the human cost of SSI, which is significant (Tanner et al. 2013).

What is infection prevention and control?

Infection prevention and control is the adoption of practices that minimize the risk of infection. This may be for the individual person, in protecting their vulnerable sites (wounds, intravenous access sites, etc.) from contamination by pathogens or reducing the risk of transmission of pathogens to third parties. Every person carries a huge number of potential pathogens and specific information about levels of risk is only known about if specimens (screening or clinical) are sent for analysis. In order to maintain practice that is safe for all, a standard set of precautions is advised for all healthcare-related contacts and this is enhanced by the adoption of aseptic techniques when undertaking wound management procedures.

 KEY POINT

Standard precautions are a minimum set of measures that protect both the individual receiving healthcare and the staff member providing the care from the transmission of pathogens, reducing the risk of cross-infection. These include the use of:

◆ Good hand hygiene

◆ Personal protective equipment (PPE)

◆ Aseptic techniques

◆ Clean procedures for chronic wounds.

Microorganisms are found both on intact and broken skin and in body fluids and meticulous adherence to **standard precautions** for all patients during all procedures will mitigate the risk of transmission of pathogens in either direction. Standard precautions apply to all actual and potential contacts with blood and other body fluids, including excretions and secretions and regardless of whether blood is evident. They also apply to contact with mucous membranes and non-intact skin.

Personal protective equipment

Hand hygiene is the cornerstone of every infection prevention and control strategy; however, the use of appropriate PPE is also a critical factor. Hand hygiene is particularly important following the removal of items of PPE, since the PPE is likely to have become contaminated during the procedure.

The most commonly used items of PPE are gloves, which must be robust, the appropriate size for the staff member, and fit for the specific purpose, which may be a sterile or non-sterile procedure. It is possible that additional items of PPE may be required and this will be based on a risk assessment of the organisms likely to be encountered and the procedure to be undertaken, where potential hazards should be considered. Plastic aprons and/or impervious gowns will protect staff members from body fluid contamination and if there is a risk of splash onto mucous membranes (eye, mouth, and nose) a mask and eye protection should be considered. Employers have a duty of care to undertake risk assessments of potential hazards that may present to staff members and to take steps to mitigate these risks. No staff member should be expected to work without access to the appropriate level of protective equipment and this is particularly important in community settings, especially when visiting services are provided.

Aseptic technique

Aseptic literally means 'without microorganisms'. An aseptic technique refers to a procedure used to minimize the risk of introduction of pathogenic organisms into a vulnerable body site, in the case of wounds, broken skin. The primary aim of an aseptic technique is to protect a vulnerable site from contamination by pathogenic organisms during medical and nursing procedures (Briggs et al. 1996).

 KEY POINT

Aseptic technique for dressing change

- The working surface or tray to be used should be decontaminated with detergent and water or detergent wipes and then dried.

- Hand hygiene should be performed in accordance with the local hand hygiene policy. The level of hand hygiene is related to the procedure, for example, surgical hand hygiene is required prior to major invasive procedures such as surgery. Providing the hands are visibly clean, hand hygiene with alcohol gel is adequate before wound dressings.

- The use of drapes and personal protective clothing will also depend on the type and complexity of procedure. For example, large drapes and maximal barrier precautions are always required

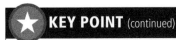

KEY POINT (continued)

for surgical procedures, whereas sterile gloves and a plastic apron and a small drape are all that is normally required for wound dressing procedures.

♦ All packaged sterile items for the procedure should be gathered prior to starting any procedure. Check that the packaging is secure, undamaged, and expiry date has not passed.

♦ All packaged sterile items, such as needles and syringes, should be opened carefully by peeling back the edges of the packaging and should never be pushed through the packaging.

♦ Wherever possible, 30 minutes should be left after bed making or environmental cleaning before exposing or dressing wounds.

♦ Soiled dressings should be removed with care, as microorganisms can be shed into the air when dressings are removed. This can be done by using the inverted sterile disposal bag from the dressing pack to protect hands or clean non-sterile gloves.

♦ Wounds should be exposed for the minimum time to avoid contamination and maintain the temperature of the wound bed.

♦ If contamination of PPE has occurred, gloves should be changed and hands decontaminated immediately. It is not appropriate to apply hand hygiene products to gloved hands.

'Clean' techniques for chronic wounds

It is recognized that the performance of an aseptic technique outside of a clinical setting is a considerable challenge (Unsworth and Collins 2011). A clean technique is a modified aseptic technique that can be used for dressing chronic wounds, for example, pressure sores, leg ulcers, and dehisced wounds. These wounds are healing by secondary intention and will be heavily colonized. They can also be used for simple grazes and when removing sutures. Clean, non-sterile gloves and a disposable plastic apron should be worn.

Screening for healthcare-associated infections

Screening for potential risk organisms has been a cornerstone of many infection prevention strategies for a number of years. This has primarily been targeted against Gram-positive organisms, specifically MRSA. Most hospitals in England had for a time implemented a targeted screening approach to MRSA; however, in 2009, the Department of Health mandated the screening of emergency and planned admissions. The impact of this and particularly the cost-effectiveness of this approach has recently been considered and the 2014 guidance is that targeted screening is the most cost-effective approach (Fuller et al. 2014). High-risk groups that should be screened include those admitted to high-risk units such as intensive care, vascular, renal/dialysis, orthopaedic, haematology/oncology/bone marrow transplant, neurosurgery, and cardiothoracic surgery. Patients with a history of MRSA carriage should also be screened.

More recently, in a response to potential threats from highly resistant Gram-negative organisms such as *Escherichia coli* and *Klebsiella pneumoniae*, it has been recommended that individuals with a history of recent hospitalization in a country outside of the United Kingdom or being an inpatient in a hospital in the United Kingdom with endemic problems with multiresistant Gram-negatives are screened on admission (Public Health England 2013).

Future problem organisms

Significant worldwide increases in prevalence of resistance to antibiotics have been observed in common pathogens found in humans. The consequences of an increase in antimicrobial resistance include increasing morbidity, mortality, and cost of providing healthcare. The cause of the appearance and proliferation of antimicrobial resistance has been increased use of systemic antibiotics. This is one of the most challenging problems facing modern medicine.

The appearance and spread of resistance in aerobic Gram-negative pathogens against broad-spectrum, third-generation cephalosporins such as cefuroxime was reported in the 1980s, occurring soon after the introduction of these antibiotics. Resistance in these organisms is mediated by broad-spectrum beta-lactamases, which are enzymes that inactivate most penicillin and cephalosporin groups of antibiotics. The genes for these enzymes are carried on plasmids that can be transmitted between different species and genera of aerobic Gram-negative bacilli. Plasmids are tiny individual DNA molecules that can replicate independently of chromosomal DNA within a cell. They can be passed from one organism to another by horizontal gene transfer, taking some of the characteristics, including antimicrobial resistance with them. The plasmids also contain genes for products that inactivate other classes of antibiotics, such as aminoglycosides (such as gentamicin).

After the development of extended-spectrum beta-lactamase (ESBL)-producing Gram-negatives, effectively the last line of defence in terms of an effective antibiotic was the carbapenem group, which includes meropenem, imipenem, and ertapenem. Unfortunately there are now significant problems with carbapenem resistance in some parts of the world, particularly Greece, Italy, and the far East (Paterson 2006). Carbapenems are a class of beta-lactam antibiotic with a broad spectrum of activity against Gram-positive and Gram-negative bacteria. Whilst carbapenems are used for the treatment of Gram-positive infections, the emergence of Gram-negative bacteria with resistance to the carbapenem antibiotics is a health issue that has prompted unusually dramatic health warnings from the US Centers for Disease Control, Public Health England, and the European Centre for Disease Control. These organisms have been responsible for large outbreaks in healthcare settings (Dai et al. 2014; Wrenn et al. 2014). These bacteria contaminate the environment and have the ability to persist (Rock et al. 2014), meaning that this could be a mechanism for contamination of wounds if principles of asepsis are not followed rigorously.

The risk of carriage and possible transmission of organisms causing HCAIs (some that are multiple antibiotic resistant) is very closely associated with wounds and wound care procedures. Utmost care must be taken in the healthcare environment (whether in hospitals or in primary care) to reduce the risk of infection by using good aseptic procedures and adhering to good practice surrounding wound management.

References

Boyce JM, Potter-Bynoe G, Chenevert C, *et al.* Environmental contamination due to methicillin-resistant Staphylococcus aureus: possible infection control implications. *Infect Control Hosp Epidemiol.* 1997;**18**:622–627.

Braga IA, Pirett CC, Ribas RM, *et al.* Bacterial colonization of pressure ulcers: assessment of risk for bloodstream infection and impact on patient outcomes. *J Hosp Infect.* 2013;**83**:314–320.

Briggs M, Wilson S, Fuller A. The principles of aseptic technique in wound care. *Prof Nurse.* 1996;**11**:805–808, 810.

Broex EC, Van Asselt AD, Bruggeman CA, *et al.* Surgical site infections: how high are the costs? *J Hosp Infect.* 2009;**72**:193–201.

Dai Y, Zhang C, Ma X, *et al.* Outbreak of carbapenemase-producing Klebsiella pneumoniae neurosurgical site infections associated with a contaminated shaving razor used for preoperative scalp shaving. *Am J Infect Control.* 2014;**42**(7):805–806.

Fuller C, Robotham J, Savage J, *et al. Final Report of National One Week Prevalence Audit of MRSA Screening.* Available from: http://www.idrn.org/audit.php

Health Protection Agency. *Surveillance of Surgical Site Infections in NHS Hospitals in England, 2010/2011.* London: Health Protection Agency; 2011.

Health Protection Agency. *English National Point Prevalence Survey on Healthcare-associated Infections and Antimicrobial Use, 2011: Preliminary Data.* London: Health Protection Agency; 2012.

Mahida N, Beal A, Trigg D, et al. Outbreak of invasive group A streptococcus infection: contaminated patient curtains and cross-infection on an ear, nose and throat ward. *J Hosp Infect.* 2014;**87**(3):141–144.

Otter JA, Yezli S, French GL. The role played by contaminated surfaces in the transmission of nosocomial pathogens. *Infect Control Hosp Epidemiol.* 2011;**32**:687–699.

Paterson DL. Resistance in gram-negative bacteria: Enterobacteriaceae. *Am J Infect Control.* 2006;**34**:S20–S28.

Public Health England. *Acute Trust Toolkit for the Early Detection, Management and Control of Carbapenemase-Producing Enterobacteriaceae.* London: Public Health England; 2013

Ray A, Perez F, Beltramini AM, et al. Use of vaporized hydrogen peroxide decontamination during an outbreak of multidrug-resistant Acinetobacter baumannii infection at a long-term acute care hospital. *Infect Control Hosp Epidemiol.* 2010;**31**:1236–1241.

Rock C, Thom KA, Masnick M, et al. Frequency of Klebsiella pneumoniae carbapenemase (KPC)-producing and non-KPC-producing Klebsiella species contamination of healthcare workers and the environment. *Infect Control Hosp Epidemiol.* 2014;**35**:426–429.

Sönnergren HH, Strömbeck L, Aldenborg F, et al. Aerosolized spread of bacteria and reduction of bacterial wound contamination with three different methods of surgical wound debridement: a pilot study. *J Hosp Infect.* 2013;**85**:112–117.

Tanner J, Khan D, Aplin C, et al. Post-discharge surveillance to identify colorectal surgical site infection rates and related costs. *J Hosp Infect.* 2009;**72**:243–250.

Tanner J, Padley W, Davey S, et al. Patient narratives of surgical site infection: implications for practice. *J Hosp Infect.* 2013;**83**:41–45.

Unsworth J, Collins J. Performing an aseptic technique in a community setting: fact or fiction? *Prim Health Care Res Dev.* 2011;**12**:42–51.

Wrenn C, O'Brien D, Keating D, et al. Investigation of the first outbreak of OXA-48-producing Klebsiella pneumoniae in Ireland. *J Hosp Infect.* 2014;**87**:41–46.

Chapter 10

Treatment strategies for wound infection

Jacqui Fletcher, Keith Harding, and Alastair Richards

Objectives

On completing this chapter you should have knowledge and understanding of:

1 Clinical features that help to diagnose wound infection
2 The difference between wound colonization and wound infection
3 The role of debridement in reducing bioburden
4 When to use systemic antibiotics and topical antimicrobial agents.

Management of wound infection

Wound infection

Wound infection is a term that covers a spectrum from colonization of a wound, local infection, to severe spreading infection with associated systemic inflammatory response syndrome (SIRS). This spectrum of severity requires different approaches to investigation and management and often treatment will have to be commenced based on the information available at the time and may have to be changed as microbiology results become available. The diagnosis of infection is often more challenging in chronic wounds and therefore the role of systemic antibiotics is less clear. If antibiotics are indicated, then broad-spectrum cover is likely to be more successful (Bowler 2002). Diagnosis of wound infection in an acute wound (e.g. trauma, bite, and surgical site infection (SSI)) can be relatively straightforward, both clinically and microbiologically. Often, a single organism (most commonly *Staphylococcus aureus*) will cause overt signs of infection characterized by cellulitis, purulent discharge, pain, heat, and occasionally dehiscence with pus. These acute wound infections are often resolved with good wound management (such as appropriate cleaning, debridement, and antimicrobial dressing) and systemic antibiotic cover following diagnosis by the microbiology laboratory. Antibiotic treatment will depend upon local antibiotic policies, as the most appropriate antibiotic will depend upon the sensitivity provided by the laboratory and will differ depending upon the identification of the organism. Diagnosis of infection in chronic or complex wounds is not straightforward and laboratory data do not always help with decision-making when choosing antimicrobial treatment, especially as there is often a heavy growth of mixed organisms with differing antibiotic sensitivity patterns. Often these organisms exist as biofilms in chronic wounds (see Chapter 6) and unless the patient is showing signs of cellulitis or systemic involvement then antibiotics do not always penetrate the biofilm. In these cases, good wound management is essential; topical cleansing, debridement, and a good antimicrobial dressing will reduce the bioburden and if there is systemic involvement, then broad-spectrum antibiotic cover is essential to prevent further invasion and possible development of bacteraemia and potentially sepsis. Quantitative analysis of microbial load in wounds has allowed prediction of delayed healing or infection in clinical studies although it is of limited value in clinical practice because very few clinical laboratories offer this service. A semi-quantitative analysis of wounds based on light (+), moderate (++), or heavy (+++) growth is frequently reported as shown in Table 10.1 (Bowler et al. 2001). Identifying the specific microorganisms present in the wound can be beneficial in clinical practice; as far back as 1918, Wright et al. reported that a surgical wound could not be successfully closed in the presence of *Streptococcus pyogenes* (Wright et al. 1918). With the advent of antibiotics, identifying pathogens and appropriate antimicrobial therapy has become one of the key roles of the microbiologist.

> **→ DEFINITION**
>
> ◆ **Colonization** is the presence of organisms in a wound without clinical signs of infection.

There is little consensus, however, about the most appropriate method of sampling the wound; numerous techniques are available including superficial swabbing, wound fluid assessment, and tissue sampling. Bowler et al. (2001) discuss the various limitations of these methods in more detail along

Table 10.1 Examples of observations that guide provision of relevant information.

Clinical and microbiological observation	Patient 1	Patient 2	Patient 3
Clinical signs reported	Pain, inflammation, green exudate	Pain, purulent exudate, pyrexia	None
Leucocytes in Gram stain	++	+++	+
Wound malodour	–	+++	–
Staphylococcus aureus	++	+	–
Pseudomonas aeruginosa	+++	–	–
Beta-haemolytic streptococci	–	–	+
Coliform bacteria	+	++	+
Pigmented Gram-negative anaerobes	–	+++	–
Non-pigmented Gram-negative anaerobes	–	+	–
Information provided on microbiology report	Moderate growth of *S. aureus* and *P. aeruginosa*; antibiograms provided	Moderate to heavy growth of mixed aerobes and anaerobes; antibiotic coverage for both aerobes and anaerobes required	Light growth of mixed aerobes including beta-haemolytic streptococci; leucocytes indicate early signs of infection; topical antiseptic recommended

–= no growth/malodour; += light growth/minimal malodour or leucocytes; ++= moderate growth/malodour or leucocytes; +++= heavy growth/offensive odour or numerous leucocytes.

Adapted from Bowler PG, Duerden BI, and Armstrong DG. Wound microbiology and associated approaches to wound management. *Clinical Microbiology Reviews*, Volume 14, Issue 2, pp. 244–69, doi: 10.1128/CMR.14.2.244-269.2001, with permission from American Society for Microbiology, Copyright © 2001 American Society for Microbiology.

with the impact of the transport and processing of the samples on the results. These methods of sampling and processing are described in detail in Chapter 3 of this book.

It is vital that any microbiology results (e.g. Gram stain, culture, and antibiograms) are interpreted along with the clinical picture before deciding on treatment. Table 10.1 from Bowler et al. (2001) illustrates this point with hypothetical examples.

Types of wounds

Wounds are described in many ways, such as their underlying pathophysiology (e.g. diabetic foot ulcer) or their perceived potential to heal (e.g. non-healing or chronic wounds). For most wounds, the most important aspect of their treatment is to remove or, if that is not possible, minimize the cause, so for a burn the immediate first aid is to remove heat from the area by immersion in cold water for 20 minutes, and for a pressure ulcer the main treatment would be to remove the cause of the pressure. Once these factors have been addressed, the majority of the direct wound care is similar and based on managing the presenting tissue type. There may be a need, however, to identify wounds at greater risk of infection, for example, trauma related to a bite or any wound in a patient that is immunocompromised, and these wounds may be treated with prophylactic antimicrobials.

The generic signs and symptoms of infection apply to all wound aetiologies but signs and symptoms that relate more specifically to individual wound types have been identified using a Delphi technique (Cutting et al. 2005) (Figure 10.1).

Surgical site infection

There are between 187 and 281 million surgical procedures performed each year worldwide and SSI has been identified as the third most commonly reported nosocomial infection (Gillespie et al. 2012). Leaper et al. (2004) identified that the range of SSI rates (1.5–20%) varied considerably across Europe as a possible consequence of inconsistencies in data collection methods, surveillance criteria, and wide variations in the surgical procedures investigated. Management of surgical wounds in the pre-, peri-, and postoperative periods to reduce the rate of SSI has been widely investigated and summarized in national guidance such as the National Institute of Health and Care Excellence (NICE) clinical guidelines (NICE 2008).

There is much debate concerning the postoperative management strategies which could be implemented to reduce these rates with, for example, the Joanna Briggs Institute reviewing the reduction of the rate of SSI

ACUTE WOUNDS – PRIMARY

Cellulitis
Pus/abscess

Delayed healing
Erythema ± induration
Haemopurulent exudate
Malodour
Seropurulent exudate
Wound breakdown/enlargement

Increase in local skin temperature
Oedema
Serous exudate with erythema
Swelling with increase in exudate volume
Unexpected pain/tenderness

ACUTE WOUNDS – SECONDARY

Cellulitis
Pus/abscess

Delayed healing
Erythema ± induration
Haemopurulent exudate
Increase in exudate volume
Malodour
Pocketing
Seropurulent exudate
Wound breakdown/enlargement

Discolouration
Friable granulation tissue that bleeds easily
Increase in local skin temperature
Oedema
Unexpected pain/tenderness

DIABETIC FOOT ULCERS

Cellulitis
Lymphangitis
Phlegmon
Purulent exudate
Pus/abscess

Crepitus in the joint
Erythema
Fluctuation
Increase in exudate volume
Induration
Localised pain in a normally asensate foot
Malodour
Probes to bone
Unexpected pain/tenderness

Blue-black discolouration and haemorrhage (halo)
Bone or tendon becomes exposed at base of ulcer
Delayed/arrested wound healing despite offloading and debridement
Deterioration of the wound
Friable granulation tissue that bleeds easily
Local oedema
Sinuses develop in an ulcer
Spreading necrosis/gangrene
Ulcer base changes from healthy pink to yellow or grey

ARTERIAL LEG ULCERS

Cellulitis
Pus/abscess

Change in colour/viscosity of exudate
Change in wound bed colour*
Crepitus
Deterioration of wound
Dry necrosis turning wet
Increase in local skin temperature
Lymphangitis
Malodour
Necrosis – new or spreading

Erythema
Erythema in peri-ulcer tissue – persists with leg elevation
Fluctuation
Increase in exudate volume
Increase in size in a previously healing ulcer
Increased pain
Ulcer breakdown
* black for aerobes, bright red for Streptococcus, green for Pseudomonas

VENOUS LEG ULCERS

Cellulitis

Delayed healing despite appropriate compression therapy
Increase in local skin temperature
Increase in ulcer pain/change in nature of pain
Newly formed ulcers within inflamed margins of pre-existing ulcers
Wound bed extension within inflamed margins

Discolouration eg dull, dark brick red
Friable granulation tissue that bleeds easily
Increase in exudate viscosity
Increase in exudate volume
Malodour
New onset dusky wound hue
Sudden appearance/increase in amount of slough
Sudden appearance of necrotic black spots
Ulcer enlargement

PRESSURE ULCER

Cellulitis

Change in nature of pain
Crepitus
Increase in exudate volume
Pus
Serous exudate with inflammation
Spreading erythema
Viable tissues become sloughy
Warmth in surrounding tissues
Wound stops healing despite relevant measures

Enlarging wound despite pressure relief
Erythema
Friable granulation tissue that bleeds easily
Malodour
Oedema

BURNS – PARTIAL-THICKNESS

Cellulitis
Ecthyma gangrenosum

Black/dark brown focal areas of discolouration in burn
Erythema
Haemorrhagic lesions in subcutaneous tissue of burn wound or surrounding skin
Malodour
Spreading peri-burn erythema (purplish discolouration or oedema)
Unexpected increase in wound breadth
Unexpected increase in wound depth

Discolouration
Friable granulation tissue that bleeds easily
Sub-eschar pus/abscess formation
Increased fragility of skin graft
Increase in exudate volume
Increase in local skin temperature
Loss of graft
Oedema
Onset of pain in previously pain-free burn
Opaque exudate
Rejection/loosening of temporary skin substitutes
Secondary loss of keratinised areas

BURNS– FULL-THICKNESS

Black/dark brown focal areas of discolouration in burn
Cellulitis
Ecthyma gangrenosum
Erythema
Haemorrhagic lesions in subcutaneous tissue of burn wound or surrounding skin
Increased fragility of skin graft
Loss of graft
Onset of pain in previously pain-free burn
Spreading peri-burn erythema (purplish discolouration or oedema)
Sub-eschar pus/abscess formation
Unexpected increase in wound breadth

Discolouration
Friable granulation tissue that bleeds easily
Malodour
Oedema
Opaque exudate
Rapid eschar separation
Rejection/loosening of temporary skin substitutes
Secondary loss of keratinised areas

KEY
HIGH	Mean score 8 or 9
MEDIUM	Mean score 6 or 7
LOW	Mean score 4 or 5

Results of the Delphi process identifying criteria in six different wound types

Figure 10.1 Types of wounds and signs of infection.

Reproduced with permission from Cutting K et al. Clinical identification of wound infection: a Delphi approach. In: *European Wound Management Association (EWMA): Position Document: Identifying criteria for wound infection*. London: MEP Ltd, 2005, http://ewma.org/fileadmin/user_upload/EWMA/pdf/Position_Documents/2005__Wound_Infection_/English_pos_doc_final.pdf, accessed 01 Apr. 2015. Copyright © 2005 European Wound Management Association, London, UK. Available from: http://www.woundsinternational.com/other-resources/view/identifying-criteria-for-wound-infection.

and subsequent wound dehiscence using negative pressure wound therapy (Sandy-Hodgetts and Watts 2013). However, in many instances SSI relates to more pragmatic issues connected to the patient's body weight, nutritional status, and presence of diseases such as diabetes which increase the likelihood of these complications occurring. Also thought to be important are patient levels of perfusion, oxygenation, and temperature during and immediately following the operative period (Leaper 2010).

 FACT

Appropriate care during the pre-, peri-, and postoperative periods are the most important factors in preventing SSI. Guidance is available from NICE (2008).

Local wound management may improve outcomes but in a more limited way; the effect of dressings is more likely to manage symptoms of infection such as high levels of exudate, and to prevent peri-wound skin damage such as blisters and skin stripping. There are little available data on the incidence of infection in other wound aetiologies apart from burns and diabetic foot ulceration.

A Cochrane review (Barajas-Nava et al. 2013) identified a limited volume and quality of evidence to support the prophylactic use of antibiotics but identified that topical silver sulfadiazine is associated with a significant increase in rate of burn wound infection and increased length of hospital stay compared with dressings or skin substitutes; however, the review authors caution that the evidence supporting these findings is unclear or at a high risk of bias.

Recent International Best Practice Guidelines (2013) suggest that between 56% and 58% of patients attending diabetic foot clinics had clinically infected wounds which increased both the risk of hospitalization and that of lower extremity amputation by up to 155 times compared to non-diabetic patients. The guidance emphasizes the importance of starting treatment early to prevent progression to severe and limb-threatening infection and thereby reducing the likelihood of amputation. The guidelines provide clear guidance for management should the ulcer become infected (see Box 10.1). In venous leg ulceration, there is little evidence that the use of systemic antibiotics has a role other than in management of clinical infection (O'Meara et al. 2014). There is some evidence to support the use of topical cadexomer iodine but according to the Cochrane review, current evidence does not support the routine use of honey- or silver-based products. In addition, it suggests

> ### Box 10.1 Management of infected diabetic foot ulcer from International Best Practice Guidelines
>
> ## Ulcer becomes infected
>
> AIM: Prevent life- or limb-threatening complications
>
> 1 For superficial (mild) infections—treat with systemic antibiotics and consider topical antimicrobials in selected cases.
>
> 2 For deep (moderate or severe) infections—treat with appropriately selected empiric systemic antibiotics, modified by the results of culture and sensitivity reports.
>
> 3 Offload pressure correctly and optimize glycaemic control for diabetes management.
>
> 4 Consider therapy directed at biofilm in wounds that are slow to heal.
>
> Reproduced with permission from Wounds International, *International Best Practice Guidelines: Wound Management in Diabetic Foot Ulcers* (London: Wounds International, 2013), http://www.woundsinternational.com/media/issues/673/files/content_10803.pdf, accessed 01 May 2015. Copyright © 2013 Wounds International.

that good quality research is required before definitive conclusions can be drawn about the effectiveness of povidone-iodine, peroxide-based preparations, ethacridine lactate, chloramphenicol, framycetin, mupirocin, ethacridine, or chlorhexidine in healing venous leg ulceration (O'Meara et al. 2014).

Antimicrobials for infected wounds

The use of topical antiseptics fell out of favour in the 1980s following the publication of key papers suggesting that many of the agents used had a deleterious effect on cell division during wound healing (Brennan and Leaper 1985). Since then, only a limited number of topical antiseptics are recommended because of associated toxic effects. Agents such as potassium permanganate and acetic acid are no longer used except in exceptional circumstances. There is limited availability of topical antiseptics including chlorhexidine, iodine, silver, polyhexamethylene biguanide (PHMB), and octenidine which are used within dressings, ointments, cleansing, and soaks. Other natural antimicrobials have been used for centuries, for example, honey, and the introduction of medicinal grade honey in recent years has seen its acceptance for controlling exudate and malodorous wounds.

In addition, the use of topical antibiotics is discouraged because of the development of antibiotic resistance and the European Wound Management

Association (EWMA) (Gottrup et al. 2013) suggests that there is an urgent need to develop an antimicrobial treatment regimen that does not include antibiotics.

Other products which claim bacterial binding action (and therefore a reduction in the bioburden) include dialkylcarbamoyl chloride (DACC), a hydrophobic coating to reduce the bacterial load in the wound, which has recently been introduced (Probst et al. 2012).

The EWMA (Gottrup et al. 2013) has produced a consensus document which outlines and discusses four key areas of controversy in topical antimicrobial use:

◆ Treatment

◆ The patient's perspective

◆ Organization of care

◆ Economics.

The document is very theoretical and does not offer any pragmatic solutions or assist in decision-making when debating the appropriate use of an antimicrobial or indeed selecting the correct agent to use for wound infection. In reality, many clinicians choose the antimicrobial dressing based on the carrier product (e.g. a hydrofiber) as they seek to manage the presenting symptoms of the wound in addition to reducing the bioburden. Sensible advice and guidance is offered in the Best Practice Statement on the use of topical antimicrobials in wound care (Wounds UK 2013). A decision-making algorithm is included within this and is shown in Figure 10.2.

Antibiotics in wound management

The use of antibiotics in wound management is not without controversy. The threat of antibiotic resistance in recent times has put an increased focus on the role of antibiotics and measures have been put in place to try and ensure their appropriate use. Whilst the main purpose of antibiotics is the treatment of infection, it has been reported that prophylactic use of antibiotics in surgical practice accounts for up to half of the antibiotics used (Periti et al. 1998). Guidance, such as that produced by NICE (2008), has sought to limit their prophylactic use in surgical practice by stratifying the risk of the procedure—clean surgical procedures, such as most elective orthopaedic procedures, require no antibiotic prophylaxis, whilst those at risk of contamination, such as colorectal procedures, warrant broad-spectrum prophylaxis.

The European Pressure Ulcer Advisory Panel (EPUAP) suggests that antibiotics are not indicated in pressure ulcers that exhibit only clinical signs of local infection (EPUAP 2009). In the absence of advancing cellulitis, bacteraemia,

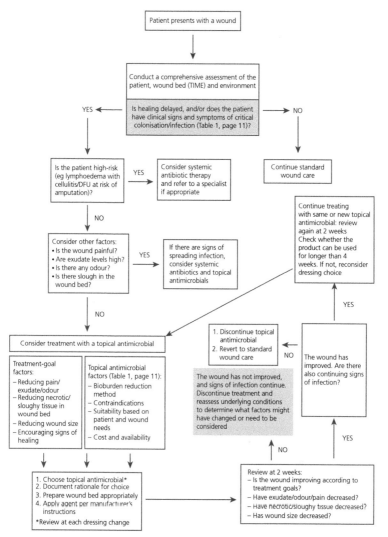

Figure 10.2 Decision-making algorithm.

Reproduced with permission from Wounds UK, *Best Practice Statement: The use of topical antimicrobial agents in wound management* (London: Wounds UK, 2013), http://www.wounds-uk.com/pdf/content_10964.pdf, accessed 01 Apr. 2015. Copyright © 2013 Wounds UK.

fever, or pain, the same principles could probably be applied to other chronic wounds such as leg ulcers and diabetic foot ulcers. The nature of a chronic wound means that there is poor tissue perfusion at the wound bed, resulting in the likelihood of poor systemic antibiotic delivery (Schulz et al. 2003; Hernandez 2006). Topical antiseptics are likely to be more effective at controlling local infection as they are supplied at a high concentration at the site (Bowler et al. 2001) and avoid systemic allergic reactions (Bikowski 1999). Others argue that due to the complexity of the wound environment, a combination of topical and systemic antimicrobials should be used (Siddiqui and Bernstein 2010).

Debridement and cleansing

Debridement and cleansing have important roles to play in the management and prevention of infections of wounds. Although defined as separate techniques (Strohal 2013), there is clearly some overlap between the two in practice. Cleansing is defined by the EWMA as the removal of loose waste and foreign material and it is seen as a separate act to debridement which can be defined as the removal of necrotic, infected, or damaged tissue from a wound until the surrounding healthy tissue is exposed (Richards et al. 2012). In reality, there is some overlap between the two procedures.

Debridement forms a vital part of wound preparation, removing non-viable or infected tissue and thus being a part of the treatment and prevention of infection. Necrotic tissue can provide an ideal environment for the growth of bacteria. As well as reducing the overall bioburden in the wound, debridement liberates the wound edge (Strohal 2013), another vital part of wound bed preparation according to the 'TIME' principles. These provide a systematic approach to the management of wounds and are based on intervention in four clinical areas which should provide an optimal, well-vascularized wound bed that facilitates the effectiveness of other therapeutic measures.

 KEY POINT

TIME is an acronym for:

T Tissue (is it non-viable?)

I Infection or inflammation (are either present?)

M Moisture (is there an imbalance?)

E Epidermal margin (is it non-advancing or undermined?)
(Schultz et al. 2003).

Table 10.2 Summary of types of debridement

Type	Mechanisms of action	Advantages	Disadvantages
Autolytic	Uses the body's own enzymes and moisture to rehydrate, soften, and liquefy hard eschar and slough using dressings and/or antimicrobial products to create a balanced, moist wound environment	Suitable for wounds where other forms of debridement cannot be used or are inappropriate. Useful if there are only small amounts of non-viable tissue. Can be used in preparation for another form of debridement or for maintenance of the wound bed. Needs no specialist training	Slower than other techniques increasing the risk of infection
Biosurgical	Larvae of the green bottle fly are used to remove necrotic and devitalized tissue from the wound. Larvae are also able to ingest pathogenic organisms in the wound (Thomas et al. 1998)	Highly selective and rapid. No need for specialist training to apply	Cannot be used for all wounds or in every patient. More expensive than autolytic debridement but treatment times are shorter
Hydrosurgical	High-energy saline jet used as debridement blade to remove non-viable tissue	Selective technique that quickly removes almost all non-viable tissue from the wound	Needs specialist equipment and training which raises costs. Risk for aerial spread
Mechanical	Wet gauze applied to the wound bed which adheres as it dries. Pulling away the gauze removes devitalized tissue	Quick and requires little training and no special equipment. Capable of removing most devitalized tissue	Often painful for the patient. Can damage healthy tissue as it is not selective. Requires frequent dressing changes

(Continued)

Table 10.2 (continued) Summary of types of debridement

Type	Mechanisms of action	Advantages	Disadvantages
Sharp	Scalpel or scissors used to excise devitalized tissue just above the viable tissue level. This does not result in total debridement of all non-viable tissue and can be undertaken in conjunction with other therapies (e.g. autolysis)	Selective and quick. No analgesia is required normally	Requires specialist training of clinicians to ensure they are able to recognize different tissue types. Potential to damage other structures including tendons, blood vessels, and nerves
Surgical	Wide excision of non-viable tissue, including a margin of healthy tissue to leave a healthy bleeding wound bed	With appropriate training, quick and highly selective method of debridement. Often considered the gold standard	Often requires an anaesthetic due to pain. This and specialist skills required can make it expensive
Ultrasonic	Devices deliver ultrasound either in direct contact with the wound bed or via an atomized solution (mist). Most devices include a built-in irrigation system and are supplied with a variety of probes for different wound types	Selective and immediate. Can be used for primary or maintenance debridement	Requires specialist training and equipment. Along with high cost or consumables and sterilizing equipment often more expensive than sharp debridement (Wendleken et al. 2010)

Source: data from Gray D, Acton C, Chadwick P, Fumarola S, Leaper D, Morris C, Stang D, Vowden P, Young T. Consensus guidance for the use of debridement techniques in the UK. *Wounds UK*. 2011;7(1):77–8 and Vowden K, Vowden P. Debridement made easy. *Wounds UK*, 2011;7(4):1–4.

There are a number of debridement techniques available, including sharp, autolytic, enzymatic, and hydrosurgical, and these are summarized in Table 10.2 based on the works of Gray et al. (2011) and Vowden and Vowden (2011).

Not all of these techniques are suitable for all wound types and the method should be selected according to the aims of treatment and an assessment of the patient and wound type. For example, autolytic debridement may be appropriate for removal of slough from the base of a pressure ulcer whereas it would be completely inappropriate for the management of a surgical wound with associated necrotizing soft tissue infection for which the management demands aggressive surgical debridement (Burge and Watson 1994).

Conclusion

The prevention and management of infection in acute and chronic wounds is a complicated process and as a result it requires a multifactorial approach. Proper clinical history and examination is vital in determining the most appropriate treatment strategy. It is not simply a case of choosing an appropriate antimicrobial according to the organism cultured in the laboratory. Optimizing all aspects of the patient (including nutritional status, supportive equipment, and management of concomitant diseases) is often as important as the antimicrobial therapy. Systemic and topical antimicrobials have an important role to play in wound preparation alongside other techniques such as debridement and cleansing to ensure the best outcome for the patient.

References

Barajas-Nava LA, López-Alcalde J, Roqué i Figuls M, *et al.* Antibiotic prophylaxis for preventing burn wound infection. *Cochrane Database Syst Rev.* 2013;**6**:CD008738.

Bikowski J. Secondarily infected wounds and dermatoses: a diagnosis and treatment guide. *J Emerg Med.* 1999;**17**(1):197–206.

Bowler PG. Wound pathophysiology, infection and therapeutic options. *Ann Med.* 2002;**34**(6):419–427.

Bowler PG, Duerden BI, Armstrong DG. Wound microbiology and associated approaches to wound management. *Clin Microbiol Rev.* 2001;**14**(2):244–269.

Brennan S, Leaper D. The effect of antiseptics on the healing wound: a study using the rabbit ear chamber. *Br J Surg.* 1985;**72**(10):780–782.

Burge TS, Watson JD. Necrotising fasciitis. *BMJ.* 1994;**308**(6942):1453–1454.

Cutting KF, White R, Mahoney P, *et al.* Clinical identification of wound infection: A Delphi approach. In *Identifying Criteria for Wound Infection.* EWMA Position Document. London: MEP Ltd; 2005:6–9.

European Pressure Ulcer Advisory Panel and National Pressure Ulcer Advisory Panel. *Treatment of Pressure Ulcers: Quick Reference Guide.* Washington DC: National Pressure Ulcer Advisory Panel; 2009.

Gillespie B, Chaboyer W, Nieuwenhoven P, *et al.* Drivers and barriers of surgical wound management in a large health care organisation: results of an environmental scan. *Wound Pract Res.* 2012;**20**(2):90–102.

Gottrup F, Apelqvist J, Bjarnsholt T, *et al.* EWMA document: antimicrobials and non-healing wounds. Evidence, controversies and suggestions. *J Wound Care.* 2013;**22**(5):S1–S92.

Gray D, Acton C, Chadwick P, *et al.* Consensus guidance for the use of debridement techniques in the UK. *Wounds UK.* 2011;**7**(1):77–78.

Hernandez R. The use of systemic antibiotics in the treatment of chronic wounds. *Dermatol Ther.* 2006;**19**(6):326–337.

International Best Practice Guidelines. *Wound Management in Diabetic Foot Ulcers.* Wounds International, 2013. Available from: http://www.woundsinternational.com

Leaper DJ. Risk factors for and epidemiology of surgical site infections. *Surg Infect (Larchmt).* 2010;**11**(3):283–287.

Leaper DJ, van Goor H, Reilly J, *et al.* Surgical site infection – a European perspective of incidence and economic burden. *Int Wound J.* 2004;**1**(4):247–273.

National Institute of Health and Care Excellence. *Surgical Site Infection: Prevention and Treatment of Surgical Site Infection.* Clinical Guideline 74. London: NICE; 2008.

O'Meara S, Al-Kurdi D, Ologun Y, *et al.* Antibiotics and antiseptics for venous leg ulcers. *Cochrane Database Syst Rev.* 2014;**10**:CD003557.

Periti P, Tonelli F, Mini E. Selecting antibacterial agents for the control of surgical infection: mini-review. *J Chemother.* 1998;**10**(2):83–90.

Probst A, Norris R, Cutting KF. Cutimed® Sorbact® made easy. *Wounds Int.* 2012;**3**(2):1–6.

Richards AJ, Bosanquet DC, Jones N, *et al.* The ongoing development of a plasma-mediated bipolar radio-frequency ablation device for wound debridement. *Wounds Int.* 2012;**3**(4):28–30.

Sandy-Hodgetts K, Watts R. Effectiveness of topical negative pressure/closed incision management in the prevention of post-surgical wound complications: a systematic review protocol. *The JBI Database of Systematic Reviews and Implementation Reports.* 2013;**11**(9):12–23. Available from: http://www.joannabriggslibrary.org/jbilibrary/index.php/jbisrir/article/view/909/1496

Schultz GS, Sibbald RG, Falanga V, *et al.* Wound bed preparation: a systematic approach to wound management. *Wound Repair Regen.* 2003;**11** Suppl 1:S1–S28.

Siddiqui AR, Bernstein JM. Chronic wound infection: facts and controversies. *Clinic Dermatol.* 2010;**28**(5):519–526.

Strohal R. The EWMA document: debridement. *J Wound Care.* 2013;**22**(1):5.

Thomas S, Andrews, A, Jones M. The use of larval therapy in wound management. *J Wound Care*. 1998;**7**(10):521–524.

Vowden K, Vowden P. Debridement made easy. *Wounds UK*. 2011;**7**(4):1–4.

Wendelken M, Markowitz L, Alvarez O. A closer look at ultrasonic debridement. *Podiatry Today*. 2010;**23**(8):42–48.

Wounds UK. *Best Practice Statement: The Use of Topical Antimicrobial Agents in Wound Management* (3rd ed). London: Wounds UK; 2013.

Wright A, Fleming A, Colebrook L. The conditions under which the sterilisation of wounds by physiological agency can be obtained. *Lancet*. 1918;**191**(4946):831–838.

Chapter 11

Future of wound care

Valerie Edwards-Jones, Chris Roberts,
Richard White, and Madeleine Flanagan

Introduction to the future of wound care

Rapid and effective wound healing is a prime objective for wound care practitioners. In addition, reduced hospital stay and wound care costs would be
ideal. A new approach to wound care has emerged over recent years and
many practitioners are seeking more robust evidence for existing wound
management procedures and available products. In addition, greater phys-
ician awareness, cost reimbursement procedures, regulatory clarity, and
evidence of efficacy will improve growth and future development of these
products and ultimately achieve better outcomes for the patient.

Continual personal development is an essential element of ongoing education to ensure that any new developments are rapidly devolved to the
wound care practitioners delivering treatment. Advances in communication
through mobile devices have allowed access to telemedicine information
rapidly and effectively and the ongoing development in this area will allow
education to flourish. Even the remotest wound can be given expert opinion through the use of digital imagery and mobile communications, so that
no matter wherever the patient and the expert are, communication about
treatment options for the wound are available. With the increasing numbers
of antibiotic-resistant bacteria and reduced treatment options it would be
ideal to have an on-site diagnostic process too, so that appropriate targeted
treatment could be given immediately, reducing the possibility of a chronic
non-healing wound developing with all the associated problems.

Today, treatment options for patients with wounds include traditional, advanced, and active products, with active products being defined as those containing actives that assist wound healing. Since many wounds can be healed
with products that do nothing more than cover and protect the wound from
infection, traditional products will continue to be important for the patient.
Small changes to the features and benefits of existing dressings which will

improve product quality may speed up the dressing performance process, ultimately saving costs and reducing staff and patient time but will not really make huge differences to the fundamental wound healing process or scarring.

Advanced products promote a moist environment and are used extensively on many difficult-to-treat or chronic wounds. Substances that help provide ideal moisture condition include hydrogels, hydrocolloids, foams, hydrofibers, and alginates. Development of these products is expected to increase and grow further as the number of chronic wounds increase. Addition of active biological substances to these products or new 'smart' materials can only improve treatment options for the future. Active products including natural enzymes involved in the immunological processes such as lactoperoxidase are already available for the practitioner to use. Skin substitutes containing collagen matrices and cultured tissue cells have been available for use in the burned patient for some time and are now gaining popularity for treating a wide range of intransigent chronic wounds such as diabetic foot ulcers and venous ulcers. Inclusion of antimicrobial substances will hopefully reduce bioburden and give the immune system some added support to allow healing to continue. The use of targeted antimicrobials would be ideal but until there is a rapid diagnostic procedure for accurate identification for the microbe then the use of broad-spectrum topical antimicrobials will continue. Some of the antiseptics previously used in wound care were deleterious to newly formed skin cells but there is a range of new alternatives coming to market that are more biologically suitable to the healing environment.

There are new developments in bacteriophage-based solutions that show early promise in adding to the armamentarium of antibiotics and antiseptics. Lytic bacteriophages are viruses that infect and lyse their bacterial hosts. They were widely used to treat bacterial infections in the first half of the twentieth century, when no adverse reactions were reported. Bacteriophage therapy fell out of favour in the West following the advent of antibiotics but development has continued uninterrupted in some former Soviet countries. In 2009, the first US Food and Drug Administration-approved, physician-initiated, phase I clinical trial of a bacteriophage preparation for treating wounds was reported. A possible future scenario suggested by Rhoads et al. (2009) would be to develop a system for identifying wound bacteria and determining their sensitivity to various component bacteriophages. The bacteriophages would lyse the infecting bacteria and kill them without adverse reactions to the host. This is an area to watch as more clinical evidence is likely to emerge in the next few years.

Research into the mechanisms of biofilm formation and agents that will act as biofilm 'busters' or 'preventers' continues to gain momentum. What would be advantageous is to know whether there is a biofilm present in a chronic wound when at the patient's side or at the 'point of care' (POC) of the patient and understand the signalling molecules present that are allowing the biofilm to remain. If these could be identified and appropriately inhibited with targeted molecules, then chronicity of wounds would be reduced and normal healing processes could return as wound bioburden decreased to promote wound closure. Many of these signalling molecules have been identified and inhibitors developed but what remains missing to the practitioner are robust 'near patient testing' or POC devices that provide accurate data on the wound status and the molecules present. The nature of these POC devices could be wide ranging with the development of new biochemical and molecular techniques using capillary flow technologies and miniaturization. In addition, sophisticated imagery, perhaps like that used in security devices, may bring a different approach to identifying the exact nature and depth of the wound. When these are available and the diagnosis of wound status is accurately identified, then targeted treatment will become a reality.

Alongside POC diagnostics, new treatment options will be developed and these important developments will be threefold:

1 Emergence of products that clean and debride the wound rapidly without pain or further tissue damage

2 Development of technologies that accelerate wound healing

3 Development of products and techniques that reduce scarring.

Developing products that clean and debride the wound rapidly without pain or further damage

There has been some advancement in this area and recently a product that constitutes a soft microfibre pad that allows gentle but effective removal of the slough and debris found on the surface of many non-healing wounds has been recommended by the National Institute of Health and Care Excellence in the United Kingdom. If this could be combined with an effective cleansing agent that also disrupted and potentially destroyed or reduced wound biofilm then its removal could stimulate wound healing. A number of chemical products are already available and comprehensive assessment of their efficacy against prevention of biofilm formation and its action against mature biofilm would certainly help in the decision-making process when using them.

With respect to the major issues surrounding antibiotic resistance, it is crucial that the role of topical antiseptics be recognized. The application of silver, iodine compounds, honey, and polyhexamethylene biguanide can, when used appropriately, be of great value in managing wound bioburden, especially following debridement (Wolcott and Rhoads 2008). Similarly, the development of topical antimicrobial peptides (Weisner and Vileinska 2010)

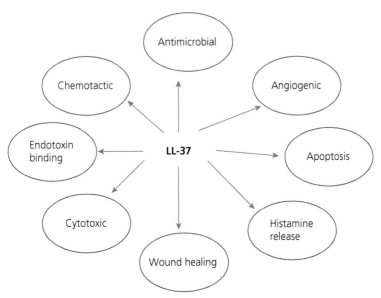

Figure 11.1 The diverse properties of human synthetic peptide LL-37.

such as LL-37 holds considerable promise (see Figure 11.1), without the risks of resistance (Gronberg et al. 2014).

Recent new products containing stabilized topical antimicrobial enzymes, glucose oxidase, and lactoperoxidase have found a large market in wound care because of their broad spectrum of activity, ability to kill antibiotic-resistant strains, and selectivity against bacteria with little or no toxicity for human cells. The enzymes work by converting available glucose into peroxide ions which are captured by lactoperoxidase and ultimately converted into reactive oxygen species which are bactericidal (White 2014). These enzymes are also shown to be active against wound biofilms (Cooper 2013).

Advances in hydrosurgical debridement techniques are also showing promise in terms of adding an element of precision to aid selectivity and preservation of dermal tissue whilst also enabling biofilm removal deep in the tissue (Allan et al. 2010).

Developing products and techniques that speed up wound healing

This area is the ultimate challenge. How do we identify molecules that can speed up the healing process and work in an acute wound environment with all the inflammatory signalling molecules or in a chronic wound with biofilm and endogenous host proteases such as matrix metalloproteinases? Molecules have been identified (e.g. vitronectin–insulin-like growth factor 1 complexes) (Upton et al. 2008; Harding et al. 2014; Shooter et al. 2015) that are involved in the healing process, but as yet none that claim or prove to speed up this process in conditions such as those seen in the patient. Other products such as recombinant human platelet derived growth factor, fibroblast growth factor, granulocyte colony-stimulating factors, and epidermal growth factor have shown a benefit to the healing process (Harding et al. 2002). Other agents such as topical insulin, topical antioxidants, and sophisticated skin substitutes are currently in use and there is research in these areas to further explore their potential.

We may have to wait some time to see products like these released onto the market but there are companies looking into this ideal scenario. Many companies look at the influence of host factors but overlook those molecules produced by microorganisms. Stem cell research looks extremely promising but again few projects are looking at the impact of microorganisms on their biological models.

Developing products and techniques that reduce scarring

In the future, it is increasingly likely that specific treatment modalities will be targeted to individuals to promote tissue repair and synthesize replacement skin without scarring. The whole process of healing and scarring is not yet fully understood but many aspects are being unravelled. Because the wound healing process is so complex, trying to find one or two elements that can influence the process is a bit like looking for a needle in a haystack. However, with the implementation of computers and robots into technologies, there are small companies who would be up for the challenge and ultimately may find out the answer. Recently stem cells with adult epidermal cell markers have been found in the foetal skin dermis. These cells are thought to play a role in scarless foetal wound healing (Hu et al. 2014). Further studies in differences between foetal and adult skin-specific stem cells may elucidate the mechanisms of scarless wound healing in the early fetus. With this knowledge, the potential to reduce scarring in adult wounds may be achieved. This research also includes building sophisticated scaffolds to replace lost tissue and to integrate appropriate stem cells within the scaffold (Larson et al. 2010). Stem cells have the ability to migrate to the site of injury or inflammation, participate in regeneration of damaged tissue, stimulate proliferation and differentiation of resident progenitor cells, and secrete growth factors, thereby increasing angiogenesis, inhibiting scar formation, and improving tensile strength of the wound. These sophisticated tissue engineering approaches, alongside gene therapy which can stimulate and regulate cellular differentiation, shows huge promise in the field of regenerative medicine and for wound therapy (Branski et al. 2009; Gauglitz and Jeschke 2011).

Conclusion

The real clinical significance of wounds, both as a cause of morbidity and as a source of cross-infection, is yet to be acknowledged by national healthcare systems. These fundamental aspects of routine healthcare must be appreciated, and acted upon. In conjunction with changes in attitude to wounds, therapeutic developments will also be essential. In the future of wound care, these treatments will come from passionate individuals who want to make a difference and can prove to the funding bodies or other governmental organizations that specific areas of research are necessary and worthwhile whilst being up against other areas of equal if not seemingly more importance such as cancer. However, with increasing antibiotic resistance and increasing numbers of patients with wounds this may become more of a reality in the future.

Finally, as is the case with all aspects of healthcare, it is vital that evidence gathered through research be translated rapidly into clinical practice. Recent history has shown that, all too often, this process is slow, taking on average almost 20 years (Morris et al. 2011). The increasing demands of healthcare systems under pressure from growing populations and limited finances, means that we no longer have the luxury of 'sitting on' potentially important therapeutic evidence before incorporating it into practice.

References

Allan N, Olson H, Nagel D, *et al.* The impact of hydrosurgical debridement on wound containing bacterial biofilm. *Wound Repair Regen.* 2010;**18**(6):A88.

Branski LK, Gauglitz GG, Herndon DN, *et al.* A review of gene and stem cell therapy in cutaneous wound healing. *Burns.* 2009;**35**:171–180.

Cooper RA. Inhibition of biofilms by glucose oxidase, lactoperoxidase and guaiacol: the active antibacterial component in an enzyme alginogel. *Int Wound J.* 2013;**10**:630–637.

Gauglitz GG, Jeschke MG. Combined gene and stem cell therapy for cutaneous wound healing. *Mol Pharm.* 2011;**8**:1471–1479.

Grönberg A, Mahlapuu M, Ståhle M, *et al.* Treatment with LL-37 is safe and effective in enhancing healing of hard-to-heal venous leg ulcers: a randomized, placebo-controlled clinical trial. *Wound Repair Regen.* 2014;**22**(5):613–621.

Harding K, Aldons P, Edwards H, *et al*. Effectiveness of an acellular synthetic matrix in the treatment of hard-to-heal leg ulcers. *Int Wound J.* 2014;**11**(2):129–137.

Harding KG, Morris HL, Patel GK. Healing chronic wounds *BMJ.* 2002;**324**(7330):160–163.

Hu MS, Rennert RC, McArdle A, *et al*. The role of stem cells during scarless skin wound healing. *Adv Wound Care.* 2014;**3**(4):304–314.

Larson BJ, Longmaker MT, Lorenz HP. Scarless fetal wound healing: a basic science review. *Plast Reconstruct Surg.* 2010;**126**(4):1172–1180.

Morris ZS, Wooding S, Grant J. The answer is 17 years, what is the question: understanding time lags in translational research. *J R Soc Med.* 2011;**104**(12):510–520.

Rhoads DD, Walcott RD, Kuskowski MA, *et al*. Bacteriophage therapy of venous leg ulcers in humans; results of a phase 1 safety trial. *J Wound Care.* 2009;**18**(6):237–243.

Shooter GK, Van Lonkhuyzen DR, Croll TI, *et al*. A pre-clinical functional assessment of an acellular scaffold intended for the treatment of hard-to-heal wounds. *Int Wound J.* 2015;**12**(2):160–168.

Upton Z, Cuttle L, Noble A, *et al*. Vitronectin: growth factor complexes hold potential as a wound therapy approach. *J Invest Dermatol.* 2008;**128**(6):1535–1544.

Weisner J, Vileinska S. Antimicrobial peptides: the ancient arm of the human immune system. *Virulence.* 2010;**1**(5):440–464.

White RJ. Flaminal enzyme alginogel: a novel approach to the control of wound exudate, bioburden and debridement. *J Tissue Viability.* 2014;**23**(2):78–80.

Wolcott RD, Rhoads DD. A study of biofilm based wound management in subjects with critical limb ischaemia. *J Wound Care.* 2008;**17**:145–155.

Index

U
ultrasonic debridement 160

V
vaccination 4
varidase 95
venous ulcers 57
  healing 130
  identified pathogens 62
  non-healing 127
Vibrio vulnificus 78–9
virulence of microorganisms 5–6, 27
viruses 18–20
  comparative sizes 4
  double-stranded DNA viruses 19
  single-stranded DNA viruses 19
  single-stranded RNA viruses 20
vitronectin–insulin-like growth factor 1
    complexes 169

W
wound care 2–3
  malodorous wound dressings 133–4
wound healing 53–4
  delayed 7
  phases 54
wound infections *see* infection of
    wounds 7
wound microbiology *see* microbiology of
    wounds
wound pathogens 67
  common examples 67–77
  rarer examples 77–9

Y
yeasts 20, 21

Z
zone of inhibition (ZOI) 108–9